How Much Can You ~~Lift?~~
Control?

**A Guide To A Lifetime of Consistent
Improvement Through Safe Weight Training**

By Bob Hoyle

For more information contact the publisher:

Hoyle Press
6707 35th Avenue West
Bradenton, FL 34209

ISBN: 978-1515011729

DEDICATED TO:

My parents, Dave and Barbara Hoyle

My grandparents, Bob and Katherine Stewart

My children, Katie and Joe

ACKNOWLEDGEMENTS

I want to express my appreciation to the following people for their support and assistance:

Matt Taylor
Jennifer LaRocco
Dr. Mont Roberts
Dr. Mark Frankle
Dr. Richard Lang
Phil Upton
Dr. Margaret Kirkland
Dr. Barclay Kirkland
Mark Scott
Joe Restivo
Greg Hoffman
Richard Randolph
Chris Hittel
Brandon Hagood

RECOMMENDATIONS:

In my 25 years as an orthopedic surgeon specializing in shoulder surgery and 40 years in weight training, I have seen and treated hundreds of injuries that were attributable to, among other things, bad exercise form and the use of excessive weight. The principles in *How Much Can You Control?* can help prevent some of the common problems people create for themselves from risky training methods and that require surgical repair. The philosophy discussed is correctly focused on the simple yet overlooked truth that the most important part of the exercise program is to avoid injury, and that training requires the mental discipline necessary to train safely. I recommend it as the perfect companion for someone starting an exercise program or someone who is currently training. In either case, safety is always the first concern.

~~~ Mark Frankle, MD
Director, Shoulder Service
Florida Orthopedic Institute

The concepts described in *How Much Can You Control?* are sensible and necessary to avoid the types of long-term injuries that require medical treatment over the course of a person's life. The message is timely for those who are training for any reason. The book provides information on wise exercise performance that needs to be known by persons of all ages in order to make weight training a positive fitness activity without the risk of injury. Bob writes from a personal experience from many years in which I have observed his passion for weight training. I recommend this book for all those who are pursuing weight training as a fitness tool.

~~~Richard Lang, MD MPH
Chair, Department of Preventive Medicine
Cleveland Clinic

The practice of Emergency Medicine has always included the treatment of people who have suffered injuries as a result of incorrect and unwise training methods. The most common problems are the use of bad form, too much weight, and the failure to recognize the significant risk that goes with weight training.

I have known Bob since our days as students at Harvard College. He has maintained his passion for training over many years and brings a significant amount of practical experience to the advice in *How Much Can You Control?* I consider it a great resource for information needed to avoid the trauma of an injury that can become a life-long disability.

~~~Mont R. Roberts, MD
Clinical Associate Professor
Department of Emergency Medicine
Michigan State University

I have seen numerous serious and crippling injuries in my 15 years of competitive lifting that could have easily been avoided if wise training methods were used. Injuries inhibit positive results. With every injury, previous gains are lost, sometimes permanently. Bob provides information that you need to know as a basis for safe training in an easy-to-read style. As he notes, injury prevention should be foremost in the training process. *How Much Can You Control?* is a must-read for persons of all ages who want to use weight training as a fitness tool without the risk of injury. Risk-free lifting is a must for achieving strength and fitness over the long haul. A lifetime of damage to the body is not worth the risk.

~~~Margaret Kirkland, DDS
5 time world champion with 50 world records and 50 national records in women's powerlifting.

I consider Bob Hoyle's training advice in *How Much Can You Control?* to be invaluable for the mass majority of us who are "hard-gainers". Unfortunately, we are not all gifted athletes. We work hard for modest results. One of the keys to the enjoyment of our lifting process and attaining the goal of greater strength, conditioning and the physical enjoyment of life is injury-free lifting. Injuries set us back and prevent us from achieving the conditioning that we so greatly desire. Bob Hoyle has remarkably good ideas to help us get where we want to be safely and securely.

~~~Barclay Kirkland, DDS, M.S.D.
Lifelong Lifter and Coach for Margaret Kirkland

PREFACE

A word about the format of this book is needed. I have written about numerous topics that are divided into three general areas: training philosophy, exercise, and diet. Within each area there is no true sequence intended to apply to the flow of ideas. I imagine that the reader will begin with the first chapter and continue progressively to the last chapter.

However, my intention is that each chapter be its own independent source of information with no real need for reference to any other chapter. My reason is to provide the reader with a continued source of information by simply opening the book to any page, and also to allow readers who want a quick reference to be able to go directly to a specific section. You do not have to recall what was written on the prior page to benefit from reading the present page.

Hope it works for you.

Bob Hoyle
Bradenton, Florida

This book contains advice regarding exercise of various types. You should consult a physician to determine if you are able to do any of the exercises that are mentioned.

TABLE OF CONTENTS

Part Two: Exercise

Part Three: Diet

Exercise Safely

Eat Wisely

Rest

Continue Forever

INTRODUCTION

This book began to develop in 1966. I was 13 and on Sundays my grandfather would take me to the train depot at Union Station in Columbus, Ohio. He went there to get a horse racing newspaper for the next day's races from the Tobacco and News Stand. I went along to get books or magazines. At some point I was looking over the variety of magazines and saw one with a weightlifter on the cover. At the time I was a pudgy fellow who participated in the usual sports, but aspired to be a better athlete. I bought the magazine and a new world opened for me. I became aware of the benefits of proper training, diet and a healthy lifestyle. I began to see weight training as a means of improving myself as an athlete.

At the time, weight training was an unknown activity, shunned by coaches and the general public. Believe it or not, it was a big deal for magazines to publish articles about football players who lifted, because it wasn't done by that many athletes at the time. Weight training was seeking its own sense of validation and identity.

I began subscribing to two training magazines and looked forward to new issues every month. I had a barbell and some plates in the basement that had been gathering dust for several years. I wiped off the dust, bought a cheap bench, and began imitating the exercise routines I read in the magazines. As I progressed through high school, weight training became a part of my participation in football and wrestling. I trained to improve my performance in those sports, but was fast becoming hooked on training by itself.

No gyms existed in Columbus, and the magazines I read were my sole source of information.

After high school, I attended Harvard College in 1971 and was around some "real weights" for the first time. By that, I mean a few Olympic barbells, a power rack, and a Universal multi-station machine. This assortment of equipment was typical for most gyms at the time. Training was still not a widely accepted practice for athletes or the general public.

My major field of concentration was biology. I began to study physiology, anatomy and the effects of training.

I taught weight training for the Harvard Department of Athletics and found I enjoyed assisting others in developing their training knowledge by sharing what I had learned.

After graduation, I began training for competition. I also taught high school and coached football, weightlifting, and wrestling. At that time, Arnold Schwarzenegger began appearing in films, and the public became aware of the beneficial effects that training can have on the body. A new respect for health and fitness was born. Gyms began to develop as a commercial enterprise, and training became a valid pursuit for fitness.

As training has become an accepted activity by the general public, I have seen many people in gyms who don't know how to think while they are there. Specifically, they don't think about the potential risk of training and that safety should be their first priority.

If I am on a golf course, my experience with the sport has taught me how to think about making shots in order to accomplish my goal in the round. Over the past 49 years, I have also learned how to think in the gym. Many people are in a gym because they know it is supposed to be a beneficial activity for their health and appearance. Yet when it comes to actually structuring a safe, sustainable workout, a lack of perspective on how to train safely and effectively can leave them frustrated and susceptible to injury.

I have seen this problem in people who have been training a short time and also those with some experience. Bad habits are tough to break. Without a good understanding of the risks of training combined with both short term and long term goals for being in the gym, training will not be as rewarding as it can be.

The purpose of this book is to provide you with information that is designed to improve your experience while training. Weight training is not rocket science. The basics are the same for all of us. You just have to keep those basic thoughts in mind to maximize the long-term enjoyment, effectiveness and safety of your training time.

Whether you are beginning a training program or have been training for some time, I provide you with information that is easily remembered and understood. I discuss training philosophy, exercise performance, and diet habits. I have tried to put some basic thoughts in the reader's mind that may assist in reaching health and fitness goals.

The information in this book is not the final word on training, nor will every part apply to all. I encourage you to use the information as best you can, be patient, and if it works, then I have accomplished my goal. I am hopeful that it will provide a basis for thought while training and assist in making weight training a lifetime passion as it has been for me.

If we could give every individual the right amount of nourishment and exercise, not too little and not too much, we would have found the safest way to health.

~~~Hippocrates

</div>

The first step toward getting somewhere is to decide that you are not going to stay where you are.

<div align="right">

~~~J.P. Morgan

You've been given the innate power to shape your life…but you cannot just speak change, you have to LIVE change. Intent paired with action builds the bridge to success. You can't just want it; you have to do it, live it…BE it! Success isn't something you have, it's something you DO!

~~~Steve Maraboli

</div>

DEFINITIONS

The following terms are part of the language of weight training:

1. Repetition (rep): One complete movement of an exercise, involving the contraction of muscle to pull a bone in one direction, and the movement of the bone back to the starting position. Bending the arm and then straightening the arm is an example of a single rep.

2. Set: A number of reps performed without stopping. If you bend and straighten your arm 10 times, you have done one set of 10 reps.

3. Press: The movement of the hand or foot so that it is pushing something away from the body from a dead stop by straightening the arm or leg.

4. Pull: The movement of the hands toward the body by bending the arms to bring something close to the body.

5. Muscle Group: Several individual muscles that contract simultaneously to cause movement of several bones. For example, the chest muscle group includes the pectorals, deltoids, and triceps.

6. Pump: A sensation in muscle tissue caused by increased blood flow producing a swollen, tight feeling.

7. Motor pathway: The connection of the nervous system between the brain and the muscle.

8. Compound exercise: An exercise that involves more than one muscle.

9. Isolation exercise: An exercise that uses only one muscle.

10. Abuse (verb): To train stupidly with a high risk of injury.
   Abuse (noun): Damage caused by stupid training.

Part One

Training Philosophy

HOW MUCH CAN YOU CONTROL?

If you don't deal with reality, reality will deal with you.
$~~~~$~~~Billy Donovan

Several years ago I wrote an article for Iron Man magazine called "How Much Can You Control?" At the time my shoulders were injured and I was becoming aware of the need for a safe and controlled manner of training.

I pointed out the difference between the concept of "lifting" a weight and "controlling" a weight, with a discussion of the superior benefits of a controlled method of training. One of the main points I made was that the performance of an exercise should never become an automatic reflex action, done almost involuntarily. Voluntary action to control the weight is more efficient, safer and is true training.

Most importantly, I included an example illustrated by a student I had taught named Ann.

I had the pleasure of teaching Ann in my biology class one year. She was a very bright young lady. Ann also had cerebral palsy, a problem which affects the neuromuscular system such that some tasks require a tremendous effort.

Writing and walking were difficult for Ann. When writing, instead of having developed a reflex ability to form letters on a page, Ann had to consciously focus an effort from her brain to her hand to slowly form the letters she had to write. She would sit so as to lean forward with her head directly over the paper. She had to see the tip of the pencil in contact with the paper in order to voluntarily control the process of the movement of the pencil. Writing

9

required a concentrated effort for Ann, rather than the reflex action that you probably take for granted.

Ann was an excellent student. What always impressed me was the conscious effort that was required to write each letter and the discipline and determination she showed in her academic success. She did not let this problem affect her in school.

As you can imagine, having Ann as a student taught me more than one lesson, not the least of which was something about training. As you become more skilled in the performance of a particular exercise, the body develops sufficient "motor pathways" such that a reflex and involuntary action is possible. This is much the same as in developing the ability to write. You don't need to worry about controlling the weight because the body has learned how to lift it and the mind is free to dwell on other things, like the amount of weight or number of reps.

Clearly a sensible poundage must be chosen that permits you to safely control each rep. Always remember that the performance of a repetition is the single most important part of your training.

You cannot take the easy way out in weight training. The natural tendency is for the body to develop a reflex pattern of movement to do the work. When this occurs, mental effort is replaced by instinct. Efficient and safe training requires that the body and mind together are performing the task.

Next time you train, imagine that you are Ann writing words on a paper with a total control over the tip of the pencil. No reflex action. No involuntary movement. Total control.

STUPID TRAINING

The glory of young men is their strength; of old men their experience.

~~~Proverbs

Elsewhere in this book I discuss the need to begin your training experience slowly and patiently. You should focus on developing the proper coordination and ability to do an exercise correctly, and avoid bad training habits.

You can get away with bad training habits for a while, particularly when you are younger or just starting out with your exercise program. However, eventually those stupid things you are doing will catch up to you in the form of injury or burnout.

I started training in 1966, and the only resource available to me to learn how to train was weightlifting magazines. I read the different exercise routines that the big time bodybuilders and lifters were supposedly doing and copied them faithfully. The articles often emphasized that the top lifters engaged in heavy high volume training, i.e. many sets and reps of several exercises per body part. There were also the concepts of training to failure, forced reps, and negative repetitions, all of which are abusive training methods. I engaged in this type of training for many years and was able to develop a physique that was fairly large in the shoulder and back areas.

Then, when I was 26, I lifted a mattress from its side and felt a sharp pain in the left shoulder. The orthopedic surgeon I consulted said it was a slight tear in the rotator cuff tendons. The shoulder deteriorated significantly over time, and eventually the right shoulder also began to give me problems.

Long story short, the shoulders became so painful that I could not sleep through the night. I essentially had a disability caused by deterioration in the joints, leading to arthritic conditions. I was not able to reach above my head for anything, nor could I throw a ball with my son. I finally consulted with a great shoulder surgeon and had a total replacement of the joint on each side.

The lesson to be learned from my experience is that my body was able to handle the effects of that high volume heavy training and stupid training style for several years. However, inside the shoulder joint, little mini-traumas were occurring over time that eventually resulted in the damage to the tendons and ligaments that provide needed stability to the joints. Frankly, I did not know any better at the time than to copy the routines that were being published.

Training was in the dark ages then, and the consequences of high volume heavy lifting and risky training style had not yet manifested themselves in the form of numerous types of injuries. In addition, the idea of superior genetics was not presented to explain how those lifters were able to tolerate that training load.

I was training then in a manner that I am warning you to avoid. Learn from my unwitting mistake. Remember that an injury can lead to a permanent disability that will haunt you forever. You do not want to suffer from enduring pain throughout your lifetime like I did. Don't replace common sense with impatience and impulsiveness.

Train strictly. Train smart. Proper form with lighter weight is always better than bad form and heavy weight.

By the way, the shoulders feel great.

DO YOU LIKE WHAT YOU SEE?

Change before you have to.
~~~ Jack Welch

If you do not like what you see in the mirror, you have a decision to make. If you do not like the quality of life you are experiencing because of your health or fitness, you also have a decision to make. You can take the steps necessary to change your health and appearance, or you can choose not to do so.

Have you become comfortably accustomed to seeing yourself appear a certain way over a period of time and accepted your appearance as an unchangeable you? Nothing could be further from the truth. If you do not like what you see in the mirror, you have the ability to make a change. Simply make the necessary lifestyle adjustments and maintain the control of your life necessary to create the change you desire. Continued apathy and complacency will kill you. Resolve to make a difference in your life. But you have to want it to make it happen.

Let me ask you this. Is there any food that tastes better than it feels to see your image in the mirror in good shape? Oh? You don't know how that feels? Too bad. Are you going to do something about it? Is it that difficult a choice?

Find a photograph of yourself with the physique you wish was still you, and place it on your refrigerator or bathroom mirror to remind yourself of your true appearance. Use your imagination to envision how you want to look.

Your body, your health, and your appearance are a direct reflection of you and the personal standards of behavior that you set for yourself. People respect a successful person because it is apparent that high standards were established and achieved. You are a product of your lifestyle habits and decisions. When you make the correct decisions regarding exercise, food, and drink, the results will be readily apparent when you look at yourself. And you just might like what you see.

BEGINNING

The beginning is the most important part of the work.

~~~ Plato

If you are in the beginning stages of training, congratulations are in order. You have chosen to adopt a lifestyle change designed to improve your health and appearance. You are on a journey that will provide you with many beneficial experiences. Training will also give you a positive diversion from the regular issues of your life.

As with all new pursuits, you must be able to walk before you can run. The initial stages of training require great patience and commitment. Do not expect instant improvement. Don't expect your body to be able to effectively perform an exercise without consistent repetition. Your goal is to safely create the muscle sense to make the exercise productive. Your training experience will soon become comfortable and familiar as you develop the skills to do an exercise correctly.

At the outset you must concentrate on developing the coordination to perform a movement correctly through a full and safe range of motion of the skeleton being moved. Keep the resistance low and focus on moving the bones in their normal plane of motion. You want to build a strong overall foundation by using basic compound movements. Always remember that the way you train is something that you control and that impacts your long-term health.

Think of developing a motor pathway from your brain to the muscle to create the control by your nervous system necessary to perform the movement through repetition. You are creating a neuromuscular groove to make a more efficient system for the movement. Remember that your body is designed to move in the manner of the exercise. You just need to learn to do it against resistance. If you use too much weight, you will sacrifice the development of the necessary coordination.

Poor exercise style neglects the muscles. Proper form is the most important goal so that you learn how to perform pure reps. The weight used takes a back seat to proper performance. Proper form creates focus and concentration. If you use common sense to do the exercise correctly from the start, you will avoid poor habits and injury.

From the very beginning of your training, concentrate on making each repetition pure and honest. Work to perfect your skill in the movement, much the same way that a golfer works to perfect the golf swing.

Coax your muscles to get stronger. Patient training is sensible training. Eventually your efforts will be reinforced with results of improved conditioning, strength and confidence.

Always remember that the purpose of proper exercise and nutrition is to improve the quality of your life. To achieve this goal, you must train safely. The body responds positively to proper stimulation and negatively to excess.

Another goal at the beginning is to improve the circulation of blood to the muscle tissue. To achieve this, keep the reps fairly high –at least 10 per set – to create a better blood supply to the muscle.

MAKE IT FEEL GOOD

A faithful friend is the medicine of life.

~~~Ecclesiastes 6:16

Training with weights should be an enjoyable experience. If it is not, you are likely to join the large number of people who quit after a few months. Your goal when training a particular muscle or group of muscles is to create a congested feeling in the muscle that you can sense when you have completed the exercise. The feeling of congestion makes you aware of the muscle that you have been working. This sensation is often called a pump, for obvious reasons. You should begin to recognize the sensation as a pleasant and sensual feeling that can be created with the correct training methods.

Train to reach the goal of congesting the muscle tissue with blood. Think in terms of blood filling the muscle as a result of your effort, causing the tissue to swell and feel tight, as if air has been pumped into it. Develop the mental ability to feel the congested muscle after the exercise is completed. This is a mind-muscle connection that makes your training more enjoyable. You are no longer just moving weight to be moving it. You are training to create a pleasant feeling in the muscle group targeted by the exercise. By reaching the goal of the congested feeling, you will have instant gratification for your efforts. It may require some time after you have started training to be able to sense it, but eventually you will be able to feel it.

Create a short term goal like "Why am I doing this? What do I want to get out of my training time? How can I make this feel good?"

In order to be effective, training must be consistent over time. For training to be consistent, it must be desirable. Feeling the pump in the muscle will make training a positive experience, and will generate new enthusiasm and motivation to make training a lifetime activity. Work for the feeling to be had from the exercise.

CREATE THE FEELING

True enjoyment comes from activity of the mind and exercise of the body; the two are ever united.

~~~Wilhelm von Humboldt

One excellent method for creating a pump in the muscle is to do your reps in proper form with a resistance that makes the last repetition difficult, with minimal rest between sets. Experiment and determine the number of reps per set that works best for you. Typically eight is the minimum and twenty the maximum number of reps per set. You won't get a pump with heavy weight and low reps.

There are ways that you can enhance the congestion feeling with creativity, but as a general rule, the most pure reps done in the least time is the most effective. Your rest time between sets should eventually be about the time it would take another person to do a set. Do not perform more sets than are necessary to achieve a pump in the muscle. I suggest no more than 3–5 sets per exercise, and 1–2 exercises per body part. Create the feeling, and then stop the exercise to enjoy it.

Your ability to create a pump in a muscle requires good neuromuscular control of the weight and good circulation to the muscle, i.e. perfect form and high reps.

YOUR THOUGHTS

Leave all the afternoon for exercise and recreation, which are as necessary as reading. I will rather say more necessary because health is worth more than learning.

~~~ Thomas Jefferson

Prior to your workout, you will have a plan in mind to structure your exercise time. You will consider options, like which muscles you will work, which exercises you will do, and the amount of weight you will use.

You have a couple of choices regarding these options and the way they influence your training. On one hand, you can pick an exercise, choose a poundage, and set a number of reps as your goal. There are two significant problems with this strategy as it involves the weight-rep goal.

The first problem is that you are setting yourself up for unnecessary frustration and potential failure if you do not meet this arbitrary number of reps with this arbitrary poundage. The second problem is that you increase your risk of injury if you break your form in an effort to do the chosen number of reps. As my grandfather would say about a variety of things – what's the difference?

Your second and safer option is to pick an exercise, choose a range of reps with the goal of doing perfect reps to create muscle congestion, and decide on a weight that feels good and comfortable on that day. You are emphasizing the importance of doing a range of perfect reps, while maintaining the discretion as to the weight you use and the exact number of reps you do.

Your thought is not, "I am going to do 225 pounds for 10 reps." Your thought is, "I am going to do 3-5 sets of 8-12 perfect reps with a weight that permits me to comfortably accomplish this goal." The important point is to be wise and recognize that there will be some days when 225 pounds might be the optimum weight, and some days when 185 pounds might be best.

Over time, your strength will increase, but you are foolish to push yourself toward a bogus weight-rep orientation that can only do you more harm than good. It is a risky and egocentric training method. Focus on a range of pure reps and adjust the weight you use to get there.

CONTROL

Men are all alike in their promises. It is only in their deeds that they differ.

~~~Molière

The most important factor in weight training, whether you are training for improved fitness, competition, or sports, is never the amount of weight you are able to lift. The important factor is the control you have with the weight you are using. "How much" isn't as important as "how well."

You must always be in control of the resistance you are using for the exercise. The proper mechanical performance of a single rep is the most important factor in effective training. Your repetitions should be slow and steady through the full range of motion. Never let the weight be pulled by gravity. Do not permit momentum to become involved in the movement by making an initial strong contraction that gets the weight moving without further muscle control. You risk injury when you are not in control of the resistance, and you decrease the effectiveness of the exercise.

It is very important that you begin each repetition slowly so that your muscle, not momentum, is moving the weight throughout the rep. YOU control the speed of the rep and the movement, not the weight. Be smooth and do quality, perfect repetitions. Each rep should be honest, with no cheating. Maintain constant tension during the movement. You should force the muscle and the mind to benefit from the entire repetition.

This technique is more productive and safer, but you may have to reduce the amount of resistance you are accustomed to using for the movement. Too bad. Leave your ego at the door of the gym. Focus on the ability to do the exercise properly and in good form for the number of reps needed to create a feeling in the muscle. You are not training to impress anyone. Numbers are irrelevant. Stay in total control during the entire set.

Never let the performance of an exercise become a reflex action that you are not consciously controlling, and never sacrifice form in favor of weight. By concentrating on the control of the movement, you will improve the motor pathways in the nervous system that control the contraction, thereby increasing coordination and enhancing the congested feeling. With moderate weight and higher repetitions you will get the rep into the correct neuromuscular groove and make a pure and precise movement. True strength is the ability to have control over the weight, not just push or pull it.

Your muscles benefit from the quality of your workouts, not by the poundage you use in the exercise. The weight you use is not as important as the way you use it. What counts is the result the weights and exercise give you.

Proper form creates the correct combination of effort by your muscles to generate the most benefit. Do your set one rep at a time. Stay focused on each rep to maintain total control of the weight. Don't waste a rep. A good rep has nothing to do with the amount of weight that is used, and a good set has nothing to do with the weight used or the number of reps performed. Tell yourself that your goal in each workout is to perform nothing but pure reps.

YOU CANNOT FLEX FAT

The excessive increase of anything causes a reaction in the opposite direction.

~~~Plato

You cannot flex fat. Only muscle tissue moves bone and can be controlled voluntarily. There is no logical reason to overnourish your body and cause it to develop tissue that has little positive function. The muscle tissue is there, subject to your choice of whether to train to provide stimulation for growth and conditioning.

If you have decided to overnourish yourself for a period of time, the muscles will be covered by a layer of unsightly, useless tissue that distorts your true appearance. The lines of your body will be defined by fat tissue rather than the muscle tissue that is really you. Muscle has a function that you can control. Excess fat tissue is not healthy body weight.

A common misconception is that weight training will convert fat tissue into muscle, or that muscle tissue turns into fat if not used. This idea is simply not true.

What would your reaction be if you were told that, for the rest of your life, you had to carry a permanent ten, fifteen, twenty, or twenty-five pound weight with you as you moved around? You would likely find it most disagreeable, but yet you are voluntarily submitting to the same handicap if you have become too large.

An overweight body is not a healthy body. In the long run, a fat person is likely to suffer from a variety of expensive medical problems. Diabetes, arthritis, and heart disease are just a few of the issues that plague overweight people. Is an overindulgent lifestyle really worth the hardship it creates on your health and appearance? If your body was a car, would you buy it?

MOMENTUM

The secret to success is constancy to purpose.

~~~Benjamin Disraeli

In the science of physics, the quantity of momentum of a moving object is measured by multiplying its mass (weight) by its velocity (speed). In order to acquire velocity, an object must be subjected to a force that puts it into motion. Once an object is in motion (has velocity) it has momentum. However, if no further force is applied to the object, the momentum is conserved, i.e. it does not increase.

So, you are asking, why the physics lesson? Does momentum relate to the performance of an exercise? Indeed it does, and it should be avoided in order to make the movement most effective.

Take the barbell curl as an example. The initial effort by a muscle to move the bar (force) creates motion (velocity) in the bar (weight) which imparts momentum to the movement. If initial force has been too strong to begin the rep, perhaps even a jerky movement, momentum will cause the weight to move without further force being applied to it. In other words, the initial forceful contraction moved the bar, but then the momentum of the bar took over and supplied further movement.

When the force is taken out of the equation, you are left with just velocity and weight (momentum). If there is no further force being applied to the bar, how effective is the exercise for the muscle? Not much. In fact, the muscle has effectively been taken out of the movement of the bar because force is not required to move the weight. The weight is moving by itself.

Is this an effective way to train? Not hardly. But you will often see people training in this manner, moving weight by momentum rather than a continuous force applied by the muscle. The tension is on the muscle for only a small part of the possible range of movement, thereby creating less work and less effect.

Consider a bike ride. When you ride a bike on a flat road, you must make an initial muscular effort to get the bike moving, after which you can coast along with little further muscular effort to make the bike move. Momentum has taken over the task of causing the movement. Now think about riding the bike up a long, steady incline from a dead stop at the bottom. Due to the pull of gravity, you cannot generate the force to create momentum. You have to apply force constantly to keep the bike moving. A continued effort of your muscles is required to move the weight of you and the bike up the hill.

Take momentum out of the exercise. Do each rep slowly and deliberately. Don't coast through a rep. CONTROL the weight by maintaining a constant force to move it. Do not think that using more weight is effective if you are not doing the work. Start each rep slowly and maintain the continued effort during the rep. Do each rep at a pace that permits you to stop it at any time. You should consider this concept as an inverse equation: minimize momentum = maximize tension. Momentum is one of Newton's laws of motion, but it has no place in your training.

PRESERVE YOUR LIFE

Health, Health!
The blessings of the rich!
The riches of the poor!
Who can buy thee at too dear a rate, since there is no
enjoying the world without thee.

~~~Ben Johnson

Live a lifestyle that is designed to preserve your life. This is such a sensible principle but one that is rarely followed. The quality of your life is defined by your health and well-being. It is not that difficult to have the habits that maintain and safeguard your health. Why would you want to live otherwise? Why would you want to live a lifestyle that can only lead to the decomposition of your quality of life and health?

What would you do if early on in your life someone dictated to you that you were required to live a self-destructive lifestyle of overindulgence, leading to poor health and appearance? What if you could see the results of such a lifestyle beforehand? What if you were shown the type of body you would eventually have or the health problems you would have based upon that lifestyle? Would your reaction be acquiescence or indignation? If you would be indignant at being ordered to live a destructive lifestyle, then why would you choose it for yourself voluntarily? Are you living to preserve your life?

There is little doubt that people who are overweight will suffer more health problems as they age than people who keep themselves fit. This fact leads to other life issues. Expensive medical treatment, costly medications with unknown side effects, lost income, poor quality of life, and numerous other effects of obesity and poor lifestyle habits manifest themselves as time progresses. It just does not pay to overnourish your body. You will not be preserving your life.

SELF-RESTRAINT

*A smart man makes a mistake, learns from it and never
makes it again. But a wise man finds a smart man and
learns from him how to avoid the mistake altogether.*

~~~Roy H. Williams

You never know the long-term effects of what you are
doing until you see its results.

One of the most difficult parts of training is self
restraint, i.e. curbing your enthusiasm so you avoid training
in a manner that has the potential for long-term abuse to
your body. I began training in 1966 at the age of 13, and as
I became bigger and stronger, the "Superman" factor began
to dominate my thinking process about my training. At that
time I did not know many other people who trained, and I
certainly did not know anyone older than I was who had
enough training experience to advise me on the future
consequences of my training methods. Had I been so
blessed I might have trained differently and avoided two
shoulder replacement surgeries when I was 52 years old.

My desire to be bigger and stronger led me to train in a
manner that did more harm than good, although I did not
know it at the time. As I mentioned elsewhere in this book,
the only sources of training information at that time were
weightlifting magazines that emphasized the heavy, long,
abusive workouts of the "champions" and made me think
that such a method was the only way to train. Nothing was
ever written about the fact that the "champions" had
superior genetics and other benefits that made them better
able to handle that training and build those physiques, nor

did the magazines ever write about the injuries suffered by others not so blessed.

Training is a great activity, but you need to keep your desire within the parameters of common sense and moderation. Be wise. You can and will injure yourself if you use bad form, or try to lift too much or too often.

For each of us there is an ideal range of exercise in terms of quantity and rest. Go outside your range and you will defeat your efforts to improve. Always remember that each workout presents a boundary beyond which your training can become abusive.

The proper use of lighter and manageable weight permits proper form for enough repetitions to get a good pump. You will also reduce the chances of permanently damaging your body and suffering the eternal pain of an injury as I did for many years. Remember, the consequences of poor quality training will linger long after the thrill of a weight-rep goal is forgotten.

LINES

No one saves us but ourselves. No one can and no one may.
We ourselves must walk the path.

~~~Buddha

The appearance of the body is defined by lines. If you draw the outline of a person's body, the lines of the outline show the shape of the body. Lines that are created by the contoured shape of only muscle tissue generally indicate a fit and healthy body. Lines that are created by fat tissue overlaying the muscle show a body that is too heavy in proportion to its height. Think about the complimentary phrase, "He/she is in good shape." This statement refers to the shape of the body as defined by its lines.

Compare the lines of an hourglass with the lines for the shape of a fifty-five gallon drum. When you compare these lines with the human body, you can easily see the distinction in body types and shapes and which one is aesthetically more attractive. What lines define the shape of your body?

The way a person dresses often reflects an attempt to hide the lines of his or her body, like wearing extremely loose-fitting clothing that is not in close contact with the skin to obscure the true outline of the fifty-five gallon drum body. Describe for yourself the lines that define your body. Are you a drum, an hourglass, or somewhere in between? Maybe you are more like a pregnant guppy or a mango on toothpicks. Does your waist resemble the top of a muffin? Are the lines created by muscle or fat? If they are created by fat, are you willing to work to change them?

GOLDEN RULE

Be yourself, but always be your better self.

~~~Karl G. Maeser

Do unto yourself as you would have others do unto you. A variation on the Golden Rule which applies to the decisions you make regarding your health and appearance.

Would you have someone treat you in such a way as to threaten your health and well being? Or would you prefer to have someone treat you so as to preserve your life and your ability to enjoy it? The answer is obvious when you consider how you want to be treated. However, the answer becomes a bit uncertain when you consider how you treat yourself in terms of your choice of food, drink, and exercise.

Do you treat yourself worse than you would want others to treat you? Do you have to protect yourself from yourself? How much do you like yourself? Do you really value health?

TWO QUESTIONS

Regret for the things we did can be tempered by time: it is regret for the things we did not do that are inconsolable.
~~~Sydney J. Harris

There are two questions that highlight the difference between someone with a successful attitude and someone with an unsuccessful attitude.

Question 1: How good can I be?
Question 2: How good could I have been?

When it comes to life decisions about health and appearance, always ask yourself "How much can I improve? How good can I really be?" Think into the future and project how disconcerting it will be to ask how good you might have been with just a little more wisdom and discipline in lifestyle decisions.

Maybe you have the experience now of looking back at a missed opportunity which, but for a greater effort, might have made a difference in your life. Learn from it. How good can you be? How much can you improve your appearance? How much can you improve your health? Only you can decide which question you will ask, and what the answer will be.

STRESS AND ADAPTATION

Three things cannot be long hidden: the sun, the moon and the truth.

~~~Buddha

The circulatory, pulmonary, neurological, digestive and other physiological systems of the human body react to the stress of exercise in a manner that is designed to deal with it so that the body survives. In other words, the body has two choices: (1) adapt or (2) perish. Fortunately, the body's survival instinct forces adaptation to the stress, which takes the form of improvement in strength and conditioning.

Muscle growth and strength development is the body's defense mechanism when it perceives that it is not capable of meeting future external demands in the form of the stress of exercise in its current state. Thus, you must think of improved fitness and training as a cycle. You do the training, which places stress on the body. During your rest time the body responds to the prior stress by increasing its ability to deal with it in preparation for future stress.

The body overcompensates in its reaction to the exercise stress. The true purpose of exercise is to force recovery and adaptation by your body. It is a marvelous process, perhaps best illustrated by the simple act of running. For someone who has not been a runner, the initial effort will be somewhat difficult because the body is not accustomed to dealing with the stress. Through continued and persistent effort the body will adapt to the stress with an increased ability to cope with it through better endurance and better conditioning.

IT WILL NOT HAPPEN TO ME

*He who has health, has hope; and he who has hope has
everything.*

~~~Thomas Carlyle

People adjust their behavior based on their analysis of
the risk that is associated with the actions they are taking.
For example, if you live in an area that experiences tornado
activity, you will make decisions on how to live in that area
based on your evaluation of whether you face a low risk of
danger or a high risk of danger. If you acknowledge a high
risk of a life-threatening situation, you will take the steps
necessary to be safe and protect yourself. If you consider
the situation to be low risk, you may not protect yourself
and could have to deal with a dangerous event that may
cause injury and death. You might call this the "it will not
happen to me" attitude.

The same risk analysis applies to your training. You
must acknowledge that weight training has a risk of injury.
The manner in which you choose to train can create either a
high risk or a low risk of damage to your body. Never lose
sight of the fact that stupid training is unsafe and creates a
high risk of injury. Respect the potential for damage to
your body.

Follow a low-risk, safe training philosophy to minimize
abuse of your body. Analyze your training methods and ask
yourself if you are engaged in a high-risk activity. Is it
worth it to have an "it will not happen to me" attitude about
your high-risk training? It can, and it will. Train in a

manner that is designed to avoid injury and minimize the risk of damage to your body.

This concept is particularly difficult to understand when you are young and progressing along well in your training. When I was training as a young man, exercising with weights was effectively just starting and there were few examples of other persons who had trained stupidly and suffered serious life-time injury. Without such examples it was easy to ignore the risk associated with some abusive training methods because I had no way of knowing what might happen. I wish I had known someone to advise me then of what could, and did, happen to me with my shoulder injuries. I hope that I would have been smart enough to acknowledge the risk and modify my exercise style.

NUMBERS

Stop listening to teaching that contradicts what you know is right.

<div align="right">~~~Proverbs</div>

One of the most common faults in training is to be overly focused on numbers. In the big scheme of things, the weight used or the number of reps done with a specific poundage during your workout are totally irrelevant. A training session is not subject to being judged as good, bad, successful, or unsuccessful based upon a quantitative numbers analysis.

Do not count reps. Have a sense of the range of reps you are doing, but do not get fixated on a number. Do pure reps, in the best form you are capable of doing. Create the feeling in the muscle as a result of congestion. If you are too focused on doing a certain number of reps with a certain weight and are engrossed in counting, you are setting yourself up for potential disappointment.

When you are thinking about numbers, you create an unnecessary weight-rep goal and lose sight of doing pure reps. The failure to do a specific number of reps with a specific weight is seen as a failure in your performance goal. You may tend to place too much mental emphasis on this "failure" to the detriment of your training. Your workout should always be a stress-relieving activity that you look forward to with a positive attitude.

Do not make a number your goal. Why should a workout become a negative experience, judged by a number? Make it enjoyable, and get away from the potential negative of a "how much" or "how many" analysis. Concentrate instead on doing a perfect repetition and feeling the effect of the exercise when finished. Be glad that you have the health to be able to train, and realize that quality, not quantity, is best. Make your training an enjoyable time, not a success or failure experience.

LONGEVITY

Decide what you want. Decide what you are willing to exchange for it. Establish your priorities and go to work.

~~~H.L. Hunt

Your ultimate goal in training is to balance the desire for short term results with the need to maintain a healthy body for your lifetime. Do not compromise your long term health with an impatient and risky use of poor training methods.

One of the most important points to remember is that training can easily become an abusive practice in your life. If your workouts become an all consuming part of your daily existence, it is abusive to your life. If you train too frequently or use bad technique, you are abusing your body. You can get away with bad training methods for a while, but eventually you will wear your body out. Training should be a lifelong, enjoyable, beneficial, and recreational activity. Always make your training a wise choice in your life, and never let it become an obligation.

Often you see someone using dangerous training practices in a perceived attempt to get quick results. One such method is training to failure, i.e. until no further movement of the weight is possible. One problem with this habit is the sacrifice of proper form. You get focused on the success of the rep rather than the quality of the rep. The prospect of injury increases as proper form decreases. You end up abusing your body unnecessarily. You might, just might, progress a bit more quickly. However, what good is the short term improvement if it sacrifices your longevity in training and health? There is nothing wrong with stopping the set with a couple of reps still possible so that each rep you did has been perfect. Again, it is an ego impulse that is tempting you. The insidious companion pulling you in the wrong direction can only do you harm.

Another abusive practice is the use of excessive weight in an exercise. Too much weight can compromise your form and abuse your joints, tendons, and ligaments. Reduce the stress with moderate training methods.

In summary, you will damage your body with abusive training that compromises longevity for short term results. You will reach the point of wearing yourself out instead of building yourself up. Curb your enthusiasm and train in a moderate and non-abusive manner. You will achieve greater results, the most important of which will be the ability to exercise as long as you want to do so.

PATIENCE

By perseverance, the snail reached the ark.

~~~Charles Haddon Spurgeon

If your intention is to decrease the amount of excess body tissue you have and make your weight more in proportion to your height, you simply must face the fact that the most difficult hurdle you face is time and patience. It took time to gain the weight, and it will take time to lose it. It does not happen overnight, it happens over time. At least you are still around to make it happen for yourself.

LONG TERM TRAINING

To keep the body in good health is a duty. Otherwise we shall not be able to keep our mind strong and clear.

~~~Buddha

Long term training is a process of self-experimentation. What a marvelous opportunity you have to create further changes and improvements in your conditioning and appearance over time.

Training should be a lifetime undertaking and a form of healthful, pleasant recreation. In the same way that you might be a recreational golfer, you should also consider your training to be a positive pastime. Learn the wide variety of training methods available and continually experiment on yourself to create new and different results.

I began training in 1966, and I have maintained the habit since that time. But, as I have "matured," I have changed individual exercise habits to accommodate the new physical abilities and needs created by the aging process. The true enjoyment that I feel now is the ability to create the same feeling in my muscles that I felt many years ago. It makes me feel like I have not aged with respect to that aspect of my life. As a result, training continues to be an enjoyable experience.

HEALTHY LIFESTYLE

A relaxed attitude lengthens a man's life.

~~~Proverbs

Weight training grew out of the physical culture movement that emphasized emotional and physical health and well-being. Always remember that your lifestyle must be planned to enhance and improve your health and appearance, and the quality of your life. Such a goal requires a balance of several factors of which weight training is but one.

Training is a part of a plan to a better quality of life and health. You should also include some form of cardiovascular exercise a few times a week to get your heart rate to increase temporarily. Decisions about food and drink are perhaps most important.

Getting proper rest is another factor that cannot be ignored. You simply cannot stay healthy and be productive with insufficient rest. Further, your rest time is when your body's adaptive mechanism is working to increase your strength and fitness.

Also, try to maintain a tranquil mind and develop a state of inner calm. The cornerstone of health begins with a serene attitude about your life. Stay calm in the face of adversity. Walk slowly. It all ties into the type of lifestyle you choose to live.

Your appearance and health should reflect the balance of your lifestyle habits. As you mature, eat less and exercise moderately for a healthy body. There is no one thing that makes you healthy or look good. Not the training or the nutrition or mental attitude or sleep. It is none of that but it is all of it. If you make your health a priority now, it will not be an emergency later in your life.

CHOICES, DECISIONS, CONSEQUENCES

But how shall we expect charity towards others, when we are uncharitable to ourselves? Charity begins at home, is the voice of the world; yet is every man his greatest enemy, and, as it were, his own executioner?

~~~Thomas Browne

I have heard people say that someone who looks good "works at it." This notion is simply not true. You do not have to work at avoiding the wrong decision. If you do, you need to change the way you approach these decisions.

Do you really have to work at avoiding a wrong decision? For example, do you have to make a huge effort to bring your car to a stop at a red light, or to avoid scalding water in the shower, both of which are immediately harmful to you? You must learn to think of decisions regarding food and fitness as being as basic as deciding whether or not to run a red light. Safety first.

In life, choices are followed by decisions, and consequences result from these decisions. A healthy and fit body is a result of a decision to choose something good for yourself, which should just be common sense. A fit body is also the result of a decision to avoid doing something wrong or unhealthy to yourself, which should be even more sensible.

You have to consider the long term effects of your current decisions. Do not do something wrong for yourself, do something right for yourself. Most importantly, learn to think yourself out of bad decisions. You really do not have to work at making the right decisions about diet and exercise, nor do you have to work at avoiding the wrong decisions.

You must be wise in making decisions. You should have two goals: wisdom – which is knowing and doing right, and common sense – which is applying your wisdom to your daily life. Do not let these goals slip away. They will keep you safe from defeat and from stumbling off the path to good health. Always remember that temptation is an assault against your self-control.

IT HAPPENS OVER TIME

Imagination is more important than knowledge.

~~~Albert Einstein

Bruce Randall won the 1959 Mr. Universe contest at a bodyweight of 229 pounds. The story goes that while in the armed service, he decided to try to become the world's strongest man. Over time, he gradually increased his food consumption by eating an extra forkful each day. He also trained with extraordinarily heavy poundage. Eventually he weighed over four hundred pounds and was capable of incredible feats of strength.

Upon being discharged from the service, he decided to reduce his bodyweight and followed the same plan he used to gain weight, i.e. every day he ate a bit less than the previous day. He continued to train, and eventually reduced to an incredibly muscular physique to become the 1959 Mr. Universe winner. His patience rewarded him with achieving his goal, and he is an example of the maxim that it does not happen overnight. It happens over time.

CHALLENGE

The only use of an obstacle is to be overcome. All that an obstacle does with brave men is, not to frighten them, but to challenge them.

~~~Woodrow Wilson

Various commercial exercise programs engage in a marketing program that appeals to your ego. The typical invitation is to accept a challenge presented by the program, i.e. do you have what it takes to participate and "survive" the activity. But does this equate to a valid pursuit of a healthy body?

A challenge is a good thing because it requires you to attempt an action that you have not done and, if done correctly, will be of benefit to you. However, when your ego gets involved, the second stated benefit is often overlooked. Instead, the risk of injury is ignored and the focus becomes the success of the act itself.

I think the focus should be on the safe performance of any program. If your common sense tells you that an activity poses a risk of injury, don't let the pressure of a "challenge" force you to do something stupid.

BODY MAINTENANCE

You cannot escape the responsibility of tomorrow by evading it today.

~~~Abraham Lincoln

The road of a healthy life is not easy, but it should be. You make it more difficult.

Do you ignore the basics of car maintenance? You probably don't forget to have the oil changed on a suggested schedule. You're likely to have the tires rotated, fluid levels checked, and battery tested on a regular basis.

Why do you pay close attention to your car maintenance? Is it because your car is a major financial investment? It has to transport you? It will be expensive to repair if not properly maintained?

Do you apply the same standards to your body and health?

The components of a healthy life are simple.

- Eat correctly.
- Exercise properly.
- Rest.
- Sleep well.
- Relax.
- Avoid negative mental thoughts.

Proper nutrition—Proper exercise—Tranquil mind

Be sensible and consider the maintenance of a healthy body to be more important than your car.

51

TWO PATHS

If you do not change direction, you may end up where you are going.

~~~Lao Tzu

Success and accomplishment do not happen by accident. You have the choice to develop the discipline, concentration, patience, and faith necessary to accomplish your goals for your health and appearance. The choice to live a healthy lifestyle should not be hard to make, but it does require total commitment. Specifically, it is simply the consistent use of common sense regarding the quality and quantity of food and drink you consume, and the activities you do for exercise.

Ultimately, it is your singular responsibility to yourself to make it happen, or, to put it another way, to avoid the bad habits that have a negative effect on your health and appearance. You must look after your own health interests. No one is going to do it for you. If you choose the right path you have the opportunity to add vitality and pleasure to your life.

We each have to ask ourselves what sort of life is best worth living and whether our actions and decisions support that life or undermine it. You may have been on the wrong path of decisions about your health and appearance, but the time exists to change the road you're on. Where do you go after today?

PARENTAL RESPONSIBILITY

Train up a child in the way that he should go; and when he is old he will not depart from that.

~~~Solomon

In the same way that you have the singular responsibility to yourself to maintain a healthy lifestyle, you also have a responsibility to your children which is twofold. First, you owe it to them to keep yourself healthy so that you can be the parent that you need to be for their support and care. Second, you must set a good example of a healthy lifestyle so they will not take their health for granted by overeating and not exercising. A child who is overweight is at risk for diabetes. A child who develops diabetes has a significantly reduced lifespan and can develop blindness. Do you want your child to have to deal with diabetes?

The next time you are in a restaurant, check out the families around you to see if overweight parents have overweight children. If a child lives with an example of overindulgent eating habits, he will follow suit because he does not know any better. Early lifestyle habits will be difficult to break.

What do you do as a parent to prevent your child from adopting dangerous and abusive habits? Is there a difference between being a glutton in front of your child and being an alcoholic? I think it worse to be a gluttonous parent because children can imitate you at a younger age than they can with alcohol consumption.

Further, how will you explain to your child when you are laid up in bed with an illness that is related to your overindulgent lifestyle? Will you apologize for not taking into consideration that your child would have had a better life with a healthy parent? Do you pay more attention to the maintenance of your automobile than to the maintenance of a healthy lifestyle of your children?

Maintain the discipline you need to keep yourself healthy through sensible exercise and diet, and you will be the positive influence your child needs for their own healthy lifestyle choices. Your child is trusting you to provide the guidance and teaching to be healthy. Teach them that health is earned. Although they may not always listen to you, they will never stop watching you. Do you want your child to look like you do now when they are your age?

BODY WEIGHT

We tend to get what we expect.

~~~Norman Vincent Peale

Do not get hung up on your body weight. Your weight is merely a number that does not really indicate much about your appearance or your health. If your immediate goal is to reduce your body size, then you might use weight loss as positive reinforcement for your efforts. Eventually, you will realize that, if you do not like what you see in the mirror, the number on the scale does not matter. Let the mirror be your guide, not a number.

If your immediate goal is to increase strength, an increase in bodyweight may be a secondary part of the process. You often hear a beginner say that the goal of training is to gain weight or "bulk up." The statement really should be that the goal is to make the muscles grow. Simply gaining weight does not mean that the muscles have grown in proportion to the increase in bodyweight. Part of the gain might be unwanted fat tissue. You should not confuse body weight with muscle. Don't gain weight just to gain weight. Make your muscles grow, and again, let the mirror be your guide.

HYGIENE

Knowledge speaks, but wisdom listens.

~~~Jimi Hendrix

During a workout you are coming into contact with numerous objects that have been touched by other persons. The spread of germs can be a big threat when you are touching handles that have been used by many people before you.

I try to avoid this risk by using a wet hand towel that is about the size of a golf towel. I put water on the last six inches of the towel, squeeze out the excess, and then apply some hand sanitizer to that end. I wipe off any handle or other equipment that I need to grab before and after the set. I use the other end to dry the handle. Soak the wet end several times during your workout to keep it as clean as possible.

TRAINING IS NOT THE END

And now, dear brothers and sisters, one final thing. Fix your thoughts on what is true, and honorable, and right, and pure, and lovely, and admirable. Think about things that are admirable and worthy of praise.

~~~Philippians 4:8

Training is not an end in itself. Training is a means to an end. The end is better health, improved appearance, and a stronger body and mind.

Do not make your training time a focal point of your life. Don't dwell on it while working or doing some other activity. Don't be a slave to your training. Get into the gym, do your workout, and get out. Forget about it while you are away from the gym. Think more about your food and drink selections in your non-training time.

Do not let training somehow define your identity. Do not let training become something that affects your attitude outside the gym, where a bad workout or a perceived decrease in strength becomes a catastrophic life-threatening experience. You have crossed the line and made training an abusive part of your life. Such an attitude is one reason I encourage you to avoid focusing on numbers in your workout. Limit your training thoughts to your gym time. Leave it there. Train to live a better life; don't live to train.

DON'T INJURE YOURSELF

The first wealth is health.

~~~Ralph Waldo Emerson

Train in a way that will avoid injury. Using proper form and getting sufficient rest between training sessions will help prevent injury. Leave your ego at the door, and train within yourself and your body's ability to tolerate exercise. You will injure yourself if you commit to a training schedule that your body cannot tolerate.

Do not seek satisfaction or respect by trying to create a temporary impression on other people by lifting excessive weight incorrectly. Don't place an unreasonable and unsafe demand on yourself to make the last rep of a set the last possible rep you can do. Do not use negative repetitions or forced repetition movements, in which another person is giving assistance to do the exercise. You risk injury training so foolishly, and you are just fooling yourself. Be safe with your form.

Injury causes pain, and pain hurts. Don't dismiss pain as irrelevant. An injury goes beyond impacting your training. It causes a disability that may affect your employment and life, temporarily or permanently. Further, the medical expense associated with treatment or repair of an injury can be significant. You will be no good to yourself if you are hurt.

Think of safe training as risk management. Recognize that exercise carries with it a risk of injury, and manage that risk by training sensibly and safely. Training in good form for a congested feeling is less likely to cause injury. Also, be sure to take enough rest between training sessions to allow proper recuperation in the muscles, tendons, and ligaments.

Avoid injury and you will be able to enjoy training as a lifetime experience. The overall goal is to train for long-term health and the lifetime ability to exercise. An injured body is not a healthy body.

Maintain a sensible and practical approach to your training. If you become too impulsive and intense, you are courting an injury. Patient training is healthy and more enjoyable. Always remember your good fortune and privilege to be able to exercise.

GRAVITY

For the very true beginning of wisdom is the desire for discipline, and the care of discipline is love.

~~~Solomon

We have defined weight training as Progressive Resistance Exercise. Think about the elements of Resistance. What is resisting the movement of your body? Gravity.

Gravity can be your friend or your foe in your training. If your idea of a repetition is to simply move the weight in any manner possible, then gravity is your foe. You are simply fighting the pull of gravity against the weight.

On the other hand, if you work with gravity by performing a perfect repetition, then gravity will be of great benefit to your training. For example, presume you are doing the bench press. You can use the pull of gravity to your benefit by controlling the descent of the bar to the chest. When you pause at the chest and push the bar up slowly, you are using gravity's pull on the bar for maximum effect on your muscles.

The process is really simple. You want to maximize the resistance part of the exercise by using gravity to your advantage. Think of gravity as a partner or as something that you own. If you train correctly gravity and its benefits belong to you. Make it yours.

Full control of the entire movement is the only way to work with the pull of gravity for the most effective repetition. When you use momentum to move the weight or when you let gravity pull the weight down with little control, then you are not taking advantage of the most fundamental aspect of exercise.

Gravity is pulling on the weight every inch of its movement. Make your muscles control every inch of the movement as well. Use only a weight that will permit you to work with gravity in the exercise. Total control of the weight is control of gravity. Own it.

THREE BODY FACTORS

Open your eyes, look within. Are you satisfied with the life you're living?

~~~Bob Marley

Generally, the three factors that determine the physique you see in the mirror are genetics, exercise, and food/drink choice.

Genetics determines your basic body structure through bone size, number of muscle fibers, and other traits. Exercise will affect the lines of your body through muscular development, thereby impacting your appearance. Of the three, food and drink choice will impact your general appearance most of all.

It has been said that diet is 90% of the success in bodybuilding preparation. Apply this principle to your own health and fitness goals. Any amount of muscle development does your appearance no good if it cannot be seen because it is covered by fat. The excess tissue covers over the muscle and becomes the visible part of your body.

If you are going to improve your appearance and your health, your primary focus must be on your habitual choice of quality and quantity of food and liquid that you put into your body.

THREE IMPRESSIVE BODY PARTS

There are only two mistakes one can make along the road to truth; not going all the way, and not starting.

~~~Buddha

With regard to the male physique, one school of thought is that the three most impressive muscle groups from the frontal view are the calves, abdominals and deltoids. The eye focuses on the middle of a person's body, so a trim and muscular abdominal area is notable. The deltoids and calves, when well developed, create positive visual lines for the body. Keep this concept in mind when looking in the mirror and deciding if you like what you see.

MILO

You must do the thing you think you cannot do.

~~~Eleanor Roosevelt

For general fitness training, progressively increase the resistance you are using within a repetition range that is giving you a pump in the muscle tissue. Work for the congested feeling, but recognize when your body has adapted to the resistance by getting stronger, and then increase the resistance.

The tale of Milo comes to mind. He was a champion Olympic wrestler from 532 B.C. Milo was known for his incredible strength and also his unique training method. Early in his career, he chose a calf and every day he hoisted the calf on his shoulders and carried it a certain distance. Over time, the calf became larger, growing into a bull. As the animal grew, Milo became stronger as his body adapted to the increased workload. He progressively increased the resistance he was using, and grew stronger as a result. The same principle applies to your training. As Milo learned, it just takes time, patience, and progressive resistance.

EGO

I count him braver who overcomes his desires than him who conquers his enemies; for the hardest victory is over self.

~~~Aristotle

Leave your ego at the door when you enter your training facility. You are there to train your muscles and your mind, not to engage in an ego trip. There is nothing related to your training, your conditioning, or your physique that makes you better than anyone else. You should be proud of your discipline, efforts, and improvement. However, do not train to stroke your ego. You have nothing to prove to anyone.

Focus on yourself, the quality of each rep, and the feeling you are creating in your body, not on the opinion you think other people have of you because you are lifting a specific poundage. Do not devalue the exercise to stroke your ego. If you do, you are trading your own lifelong health for a temporary impression you may or may not make on a random group of strangers at the gym.

We are all ego-prone when it comes to different facets of our lives. The ego can be a sinister companion in the gym who makes you do stupid things. You need to avoid any tendency to tie your ego into exercise performance. In other words, do not become self-absorbed in your training. Don't let a number of reps or an amount of weight inflate your pride. Respect the risk that training has for injury. After all, it is only a number.

WILL POWER

A man without self-control is as defenseless as a city with broken walls.

~~~Proverbs

Discipline your will. The term "will power" means the power to control what you will decide to do in a particular situation. If you are going to succeed in anything, you must be able to control and self-regulate your impulses. Only you can determine your own behavior, be it eating, drinking, working, exercising, or any other activity in your life. By learning to discipline your will in all facets of your life, you learn to do what you have to do, not what you want to do. Take your discipline with you to apply to your life experiences.

If there is a question about your behavior, you first must ask yourself to answer it truthfully and correctly. You must then listen to your answer and act accordingly.

I have often thought how beneficial it would be to create a pill which provides a person with the power to discipline the will. Unfortunately, no drug company can come up with a chemical compound to provide artificial discipline to the human spirit.

THE BODY TRIES TO ADAPT

Walking is man's best medicine.
~~~Hippocrates

As your body begins to adapt to the stress of an exercise movement, eventually further response in terms of growth and a pump becomes more difficult. Your body wants to create a path of least resistance by adjusting to the stress of the exercise as soon as possible. When you change the performance of an exercise and the corresponding stress, the body creates new neuromuscular "grooves" (motor pathways) to do the movement. This process makes the effort of the muscle more efficient over time, but in turn makes the exercise less effective due to the adaptation.

Keep in mind that for general improved health and strength, you are not trying to get stronger in just one exercise movement per body part. For continued improvement change the exercises and their performance to create different stimulation. You are trying to confuse the muscles with the varied movements. When you change the stress, you create a need for the body to change and adapt.

Pick a few different exercises for each body part and consistently change those that you are using. Avoid the concept of a routine of exercises. Doing a routine means that it never changes. The only routine you do should be the habit of consistent training. Think in terms of a workout schedule, i.e. a schedule of the parts of the body you are going to train in the workout. Do not limit your thoughts to just one or two movements for those body parts. Take full advantage of the marvelous adaptation process in your body by subjecting your muscles to a variety of stimulations. Do not let your body get bored with your program.

INDIVIDUALISM

There is nothing noble in being superior to your fellow men. True nobility lies in being superior to your former self.

~~~Ernest Hemingway

Training is the ultimate individual activity. This fact has its good points and its bad points. It is good because each of us adapts differently to the stress of exercise. Our individual genetics and self-discipline become apparent as we progress in our training, and reward us with the feeling of satisfaction at the changes we are making in ourselves.

The negative is that some people look for only one method, or one set way of exercising to improve their health and appearance that applies to them as individuals. This tendency to try to confine training into a neat one-size-fits-me method will limit your improvement over time. There is not any single choice of exercises or performance that will always work best or be the safest for you.

You must experiment constantly and keep the body in a confused state so adaptation will continue. Analyze the exercise to make sure your body is suited to do it safely. Do not think that one favorite exercise will always work best for you. Your individuality requires the challenge of variety.

ETERNAL SUFFERING

Sin is man saying to God,
 "Leave me alone."
Hell is God's way of saying,
 "You may have your wish."

~~~C.S. Lewis

Live safely

Eat safely

Train safely

These three rules of life cannot be disputed nor can they be ignored.

What is the penalty for breaching these basic lessons? Are you creating your own hellish life if you suffer the consequences of illness and injury due to unhealthy eating and risky training?

Are there any good reasons for you to make circumstances in your life that create an intolerable existence? Do you want to have to deal with a life of illness in the form of diabetes, heart disease, cancer, and other medical problems associated with unsafe eating and drinking? Do you want to deal with the eternal pain of an injury caused by unsafe training?

I have said elsewhere in this book that you never know the consequences of your actions until something happens as a result. Decisions are often not rational or they are based upon a faulty analysis of the consequences of the choice. Each of us has the opportunity to create our personal living hell of a life through unsafe living. We have to figure out what kind of life is worth living and are we pursuing that life?

What is your answer?

YOU

Make the most of yourself because that is all there is of you.

~~~Ralph Waldo Emerson

The great benefit of making the decision to have a healthy combination of exercise and food choice is that the result is clearly visible: You. Your health, your appearance, and everything that is you are reflected by the time and effort you choose for exercise and by proper food choices.

This is unlike other activities where time and effort are spent to develop a skill. A golfer may have the ability to hit a golf ball 300 yards as a result of hours of disciplined training. However, the results of the effort are visible in only a limited context, i.e. on the course. The results of your efforts to train and choose food wisely are visible constantly as your physical being.

Your body is not the means to the end, but is the end itself. You are not using your body to achieve something, like hitting a golf ball. You are using your efforts to improve your fitness and appearance. Be proud of yourself.

LET IT GO

Some of us think holding on makes us strong; but
sometimes it is letting go.

~~~Herman Hesse

Can you describe your lifestyle and distinguish between behaviors and habits that are good for you and those that are bad for you? Of course you can. We each have habits that are valuable and worthwhile. We also have habits that are worthless and may be damaging to our health and wellbeing.

Do you find it difficult to hold on to a habit or behavior that is good for you? For example, doing a safe exercise schedule on a regular basis is generally a positive lifestyle. Eating fruits and vegetables daily is also a good choice. Are you strong enough in your sense of discipline and self control to maintain and hold on to positive actions?

On the other hand, you can certainly identify your habits that are not good or safe for you. Choosing to avoid regular safe exercise. Exercising stupidly. Eating too much unhealthy food. Alcoholism. The list could go on and on, and for most of these damaging habits there is a question as to its contribution to your unsafe lifestyle. The question you are already faced with, as you look in the mirror and decide if you like what you see, is whether you have the strength to let go. Do you have the strength to let go of something that has a false sense of artificial importance to you, in exchange for something more valuable to good health?

Are you strong enough to hold on to the habit of regular, safe, and effective exercise? Are you strong enough to let go of your alcohol consumption or your binge eating, or your lazy attitude toward exercise? Are you?

You have to be strong and let go of something bad in exchange for receiving something good. Each of us has a traitor within ourselves who tries to slide back into the well-worn ruts of unsafe living in the road of life. Be strong and create a new path of healthy living.

REST

Mastering others is strength.
Mastering yourself is true power.

~~~Lao Tzu

Sufficient rest is as important as your choice of exercises. You should put as much emphasis on your rest time as you put into your exercise time. Keep recuperation as a dominant training thought. Rest harder than you train.

Your body undergoes its adaptive growth process while you are away from the gym. The equation is simple: stress followed by recovery equals progress. Further, you simply must give the muscles, ligaments, tendons, and your mind an opportunity to recuperate between training sessions. If not, you risk injury and will not approach your training with the necessary physical and mental energy to make it productive and worthwhile.

Experiment on yourself to see what is best for you. Generally, at least two days rest between workouts for the same body part is ideal, but more may be best for you. You can often tell if you need more rest by your ability to create congestion in the muscle you are training. If it is very difficult to get a pump, then you may not have taken enough rest since the last workout.

Frankly, the more frequently you train, the less productive your training will be. Your rest days are not causing any regression in your development. When you rest, your body is replenishing the resources it used in the stress of the exercise. When you are feeling rested, your body will adapt effectively to the stress of exercise. If you are physically or mentally tired or fatigued, your body needs rest and not stress. Your body does not know what day it is, so do not stick to a rigid schedule.

You want to ensure recovery. Doing nothing is doing something good for you. Too much of a good thing is usually not beneficial, and this certainly applies to weight training. Be consistent and committed, but be moderate in your enthusiasm. Train as little as possible but train as effectively as you can. Always remember that it is easy for training to become abusive.

THE MIRROR

Problems don't age well.
~~~Unknown

Look in the mirror. Take off the rose-colored glasses and be totally honest in your evaluation. What you see in your reflection is you. Your appearance is no coincidence. It is a reflection of you and your daily choice of lifestyle and, to a certain degree, your sense of self-respect. Your body and your health are the expression of your life and the way you have chosen to live it.

Discipline your will. Do things you feel proud of, both in your pursuit of improved fitness and appearance, and in your personal and professional life. What truly is your "will"? Is it not merely the mental process by which you make voluntary choices?

Habits are nothing more than choices which are almost involuntary. Decisions you have made thus far in your life are staring back at you in the mirror. Are you satisfied with what you see? If not, you have a decision to make regarding your future lifestyle choices.

Live so that you approve of the image in the mirror. Your life is what you choose. Your mind creates your body and your health.

GENETICS

Breed is stronger than pasture.

~~~George Eliot

Genetics determines to a great degree your basic body structure and your general rate of adaptation to and tolerance of exercise. You cannot do anything about the size of your skeletal frame. A person with a large frame can carry more body weight and still look in good proportion. A person with a smaller frame cannot carry a lot of weight without it looking unsightly because it will not be in good proportion to height.

Likewise, genetics determines the leverage a muscle has: the ease with which a muscle can move a bone is related to the point on the bone where the muscle is attached. The farther down the bone from the joint that the muscle is attached, the greater the leverage and the easier the movement by the muscle.

Given these facts, just ignore them. You are who you are and cannot do anything about your genetic makeup. You can, however, take what you are and what you have and through consistent and persistent effort improve yourself and become what you want to be. Just recognize the fact that some people are by nature better suited to develop strength and fitness. Naturally strong people have greater neurological ability to use more of their muscle fibers than those with lower neurological ability. Therefore, do not make comparisons between yourself and others.

Training will develop your potential; what can happen, will happen. Train within your own capabilities and genetic potential. Each of us has our own individual ability to absorb the stress of exercise and adapt to the stress. We also have different body chemistries and mental traits that affect our reaction to stress. If you train beyond the genetic ability of your body to deal with the stress, you risk an injury that may plague you for your lifetime. Your body will be in a state of distress.

Unfortunately we do not have a built-in gauge to provide a guide for our individual tolerance for exercise. Therefore, I suggest you pursue a consistent course of moderation in your training.

MOTIVATION

Act as if it were impossible to fail.
~~~Dorothea Brande

Develop the desire and discipline to do the training necessary to achieve your goals of improved fitness and appearance. Use imagery to motivate yourself by visualizing the physique you desire. Imagery is a powerful tool. You might find a past photo of yourself with the appearance you wish you had now. Post it on the refrigerator for motivation. What you believe through the process of visual imagery you are closer to achieving. Sit quietly and use your imagination to form a visual image of you as you wish to be. Always set realistic goals.

Consistency, persistence, and patience will supplement your discipline and lead to success. You are doing something good for yourself, and for good reason. Your body requires a steady dose of demands and stress in order to make consistent progress. You will begin to see and feel results, and sense the positive reinforcement that comes with improvement. Discipline, concentration, patience, and faith are the ingredients of success. Most of all, do not give up on yourself.

CAR PARKING

To be one's self, and unafraid whether right or wrong, is more admirable than the easy course of surrender to conformity.

~~~Irving Wallace

I want to combine two observations in this chapter. Observation number one is the number of people who make the excuse that they don't have enough time in their life to exercise. Observation number two is the value that seems to be placed on locating a parking spot that is closest to the door.

I have the habit of parking far enough away from a building so as to have my car isolated from other vehicles. I avoid the risk of damage due to the stupid opening of car doors by adjacent drivers. Trying to find a spot closer to the door is not important to me when compared to preserving my vehicle.

An equally important benefit of this parking habit is the opportunity to walk farther than I would if I parked closer. Even if it is only 50 yards, it is a chance to exercise a bit.

Now let's combine these two observations. Are you a person who complains that you cannot find the time to exercise? Are you also a person who seeks the closest parking spot to the door? Is there a reason you cannot or do not park farther away? Is it that big a deal to walk an extra 100 yards?

Is it more important to get that closer spot or to take advantage of the opportunity to walk?

HABITS YOU CANNOT AFFORD

Cultivate only those habits that you are willing should master you.

~~~Elbert Hubbard

An old friend would say, "If you cannot afford your habits, drop them." So simple and yet so true.

Apply this statement to your own lifestyle habits and determine those behaviors you can't afford because of their negative effect on your health and appearance. This will probably not be a difficult analysis. Once you have determined the habits in this category, just drop them from your lifestyle. If you do not drop a bad habit, it might drop you. You cannot change what you tolerate.

Do you have dietary habits that you feel you simply cannot do without? Some food habit, some drink habit, or some eating habit? If you think you cannot do without it, you do not possess it. Whatever it might be, it controls you. You do not possess that which you cannot control. As my grandfather would say when he quit drinking alcohol, it was time to see if he had it or it had him. Do your habits control you?

Many obstacles to health improvement grow out of the relationships you have with other people. Spending time with persons whose goals are different from yours is a negative part of your life that should be avoided. Have habits that support a healthy lifestyle. Try to create an environment that supports your healthy lifestyle. Avoid negative influences that may be supporting habits you cannot afford. Stay out of the bars and food buffets. If you lie down with dogs you will get fleas. Be careful who you imitate, both in terms of exercise performance, your food consumption, and your lifestyle habits.

YOUR CAR, YOUR PET, AND YOU

Without health, life is not life; it is only a state of languor and suffering—an image of death.

~~~Buddha

Would you put sand or water in the fuel tank of your car or consistently drive your car at 90 miles per hour? Would you force your pet to overeat, or prevent your pet from going outside to move around and exercise? You have a choice regarding these actions, and your decision is determined by what is best to preserve your vehicle or pet. You have the same choices about the lifestyle you lead and the habits you have that determine how well you preserve your health and appearance. Treat yourself better than you treat your vehicle and pet. Why would you ever decide to do otherwise?

THE HELPFUL SORT

If I am walking with two other men, each of them shall serve as my teacher. I will pick out the good points of the one and imitate them, and the bad points in the other and correct them in myself.

~~~Confucius

If you train at a gym, you may have encountered that helpful person who wants to give you unsolicited advice regarding your training. The degree of "help" can range from a polite suggestion to an overbearing demand for compliance. In either case, analyze the advice in terms of whether it appears to create a greater risk of injury in light of the suggestions in this book. My observation has often been that the unsolicited adviser may simply feel threatened by viewing an exercise performance that conflicts with his or her personal opinion of training.

ASK AND YOU WILL RECEIVE

Ask and it will be given to you;
search and you will find;
knock and the door will be opened for you.

~~~Jesus

You do not possess because you do not ask. This is a Biblical verse which is applicable to a variety of human endeavors. Considered in terms of personal fitness and health, you cannot have a fit and healthy body without asking something of yourself in the way of commitment, discipline, patience, faith, common sense, and other intangibles which are keys to achieving a goal.

At some point, you have to assume the self-responsibility to look after your own health interests. Perhaps you ask of yourself, but for some reason a part of you denies the request. It can be like the old cartoon with the angel on one shoulder and the devil on the other shoulder. The angel is asking you, "Will you please go to the gym tonight?" or "Please do not eat those donuts because they are not good for you." The devil on the other shoulder answers the questions by making an excuse for not going to the gym or rationalizes eating the donuts. Maybe it is our conscience that asks us to do the right thing, and our success depends on the response we choose to provide. It is all about what we ask of ourselves and the response we give to the question.

I think one important facet of training that is part of what we ask of ourselves deals with the personal relationship to training. An old adage states that it is all about the journey. Maybe the actual training is not as important as our sense of commitment and dedication to it, i.e. our true relationship with the effort that can occur only when we ask of ourselves.

Part Two

Exercise

TEN BASIC RULES FOR BEGINNERS

Prevention is better than cure.

~~~Desiderius Erasmus

1. Train as little as possible. Train safely.

2. Give your body time to recover from the last workout. Rest.

3. Use the basic exercises to train the entire body using the fewest exercises.

4. Always use perfect form and make each rep pure and honest.

5. Progressively and patiently increase the weight you use or the reps you perform for the range of reps to get a pump.

6. Train consistently, wisely, and sensibly.

7. Eat smart. Eat less. Eat natural food.

8. Pick one basic exercise for each body part, and do 2-3 sets of 10-12 reps.

9. Do some form of cardiovascular/respiratory training.

10. Live safely. Eat safely. Train safely.

THE EGG

Self-control is one mark of a mature person; it applies to control of language, physical treatment of others, and the appetites of the body.

~~~Joseph B Wirthlin

Control of the weight through the entire rep is necessary for both safety and the best result in the exercise. Consider the following thought: imagine an egg at the beginning and end of each rep. If you do the rep too hard and quickly, your hand will hit the egg with too much force and break it. If you control the weight properly, you will end the rep softly with your hand tapping the egg gently. If you are doing a bench press, lower the weight and touch the chest softly enough so as to avoid breaking the imaginary egg. When you press the bar over your chest, don't break the egg at the top.

Do soft reps, not hard reps.

LEARN EXERCISE PERFORMANCE

Tell me and I forget. Teach me and I remember. Involve me and I learn.

~~~Benjamin Franklin

There are six basic muscle groups or sections of the body (shoulders, arms, chest, back, abdominals, legs), and there are several corresponding compound or isolation movements that will work those muscles. Arnold Schwarzenegger's book Encyclopedia of Modern Bodybuilding is an excellent resource to learn the exercises.

Do not limit your knowledge to opinions expressed at your training facility. Be careful who you choose to imitate in exercise performance. When I began training, there were no gyms available, and the basement was the only place to train. I learned by reading available materials and applying the concepts I read to my training. You should recognize that there is information on training that is intended to educate and direct you, and information intended to sell you on commercial interests.

Learn the proper performance of some of the numerous exercises that exist, and the muscles involved in producing the movement of the skeleton caused by the exercise. Pay particular attention to proper posture and body alignment for the exercise. When you do the exercise correctly you will have the success and confidence to bring you back and make training a long-term activity. Your exercise form is a part of your training that you control and that will affect your long-term health and quality of life.

Lastly, be aware that your body is unique and may not be suited to do a particular exercise safely. If an exercise does not feel good, don't do it.

It is your body. Your appearance and your health are you. Why would you not want to learn how your body functions and what means are available to improve your health and appearance?

FORCE

Force has no place where there is need of skill.

<p style="text-align:right">~~~Herodotus</p>

The application of force changes the state of rest of an object, i.e. moves it. Force that is excessive is most likely to cause injury.

Many training methods that you observe are based upon the application of high force to weight. Such methods create a much higher risk of injury. If you jerk or yank a weight with a sudden application of force, you are exposing your body to an excessive force. Go easy with the weight. Pull it, don't jerk it. Push it, don't bounce it.

There is a tendency in athletic training to do "explosive" lifts like power cleans. I believe that the risk of a long term permanent injury associated with the use of excessive force for this type of training far outweighs whatever nominal advantage in strength and development might occur from the movement.

For example, I have seen an injury in which the biceps tendon tears away from the forearm bone when a bar is jerked from the floor with the arm bent and not straight. The tendon literally snaps and rolls up off the bone. The surgery required to repair this injury is not fun and the arm is rarely fully functional afterwards.

If the level of competent instruction to perform the exercise does not match the technique of the movement, then the risk of injury is certainly compounded. My son Joe enrolled in a weight training class in high school. He was too small to play football and the football coach taught the class. The coach demonstrated the power clean exercise the first two classes and then offered no further instruction.

Joe avoided the lift because, quite sensibly, he knew he could not do it correctly and did not want to risk injury. The coach hassled him every day to do "cleans" without offering any further instruction, and eventually Joe dropped the class.

The point is that if my son or daughter was going to participate on a school team that had a weight training component, I would check the background and credentials of the coach who was teaching the exercises to confirm an acceptable level of competence.

PROPER FORM

We cannot solve our problems with the same level of
thinking that created them.

~~~Albert Einstein

You must stay focused on the proper form required to do an exercise correctly. Never sacrifice proper form (quality) for more resistance (quantity). Your muscles do not know the difference between 10 pounds and 100 pounds. Only your ego knows the difference, and I cannot advise you often enough to leave the ego at the door of the gym.

Use the full movement of the bone, from full stretch of the muscle to full contraction of the muscle. Always perform a repetition smoothly and slowly, with no sudden jerking of the weight. Start each rep slowly. Make each rep a perfect rep. An incorrect use of excessive resistance leads to improper form. Improper form then results in less pump, less improvement, and possible injury. Strength can only be measured by pure reps.

Take the time to learn the proper way to do an exercise safely. You will find that common sense prevails when analyzing movements, as they are defined by the normal movement of the skeleton. Doing an exercise with proper biomechanical form engages the muscles correctly by creating the proper coordinated effort.

Weight training is not rocket science. Develop a controlled, health oriented and safe workout with proper form. Do the exercise correctly, and you will get the most benefit from it. Make the exercise work for you.

The biggest mistake made in weight training is the use of too much weight with improper form. Excessive "cheating" in an exercise movement is wasted effort and misdirected stress. The weight is moving by itself through the force of momentum, and not through the effort of the muscles.

Get your mind off the number and into the proper performance with a resistance you can control. The more work you perform correctly within a short time, the more progress you should make.

Let the workout "work" for you. This means taking your time and doing it right.

FULL RANGE OF MOTION

Success is simple.
Do what's right, the right way, at the right time.

~~~Arnold A. Glason

Skeletal muscle moves bones through specific planes and ranges of motion, and this movement defines the function of the muscle. An exercise is simply the muscle performing its normal function against some form of resistance.

Do an exercise through the entire and normal function of the muscle group. Perform a complete movement of the bone that is being moved by the target muscle group in a range that is safe for you. Pause at both ends of the movement but avoid a hard lockout of the arm or leg when it is straightened.

PROGRESSIVE RESISTANCE EXERCISE

Shallow men believe in luck. Strong men believe in cause and effect.

~~~Ralph Waldo Emerson

One definition of weight training is Progressive Resistance Exercise.

Progressive means improvement in a defined manner with a gradual increase over time. For example, adding five pounds to the bar or an additional repetition every five workouts progressively increases the intensity of the exercise.

Resistance is the load that is attached to the bone that is moved by the muscle.

Exercise is the particular movement of a bone by a muscle, subject to the weight chosen to create resistance.

Progressive resistance exercise requires a patient attitude. You must be patient to progressively increase the resistance you are using in an exercise. Coax the muscles along the path of development and strength.

MUSCLE TISSUE

The body never lies
                    ~~~Martha Graham

You have three types of muscle tissue in the body.

Skeletal muscle is attached to the bones of your skeleton and contracts to provide movement of the bones. Skeletal muscle has an origin point on a stationary bone and an insertion point on the bone that it moves. Skeletal muscle gives a body its shape and contour (lines). This type of muscle is subject to voluntary contractions and moves a bone by shortening its length in the contraction process.

Cardiac muscle is the heart muscle tissue. Cardiac muscle contracts like a fist to force blood throughout the body through arteries and veins. The heart is capable of contracting more frequently and with greater stroke volume to accommodate a need for increased blood flow to the body due to oxygen depletion from exercise.

Smooth muscle tissue makes up the digestive system, extending from the esophagus to the colon as one continuous tube. Smooth muscle contracts involuntarily in response to the presence of food by squeezing in a wave effect called peristalsis that pushes food through the tube for breakdown and eventual absorption.

WARM UP SETS

Do or do not. There is no try.

~~~Yoda

It is beneficial to begin an exercise with light warm up sets. These sets get the connection between the mind and muscle primed and ready to feel the effect of the exercise. You might think of warm up sets in the same manner as a golfer takes practice swings before a shot.

Your first set of an exercise should be with a very light resistance for numerous repetitions. If you are doing an exercise with a bar, use just the bar in the exercise motion. Do the reps smoothly and perfectly to get the muscle and joint fully stretched and to warm up the neuromuscular pathway between the brain and the muscle to prepare for the mental coordination of the movement. You are creating a "groove" in your coordination for the exercise to remind your body how to do the movement. This groove is necessary to perform the movement safely.

The warm up sets "wake up" the muscle, the nervous system, and the circulatory system, leading to better stimulation in the subsequent work sets. Do not limit yourself to just one warm up set. Be patient. Tolerate your body's need to be adequately prepared. There is nothing wrong with doing a couple of warm up sets. Perform the reps slowly and with perfect form to get the groove functioning correctly and comfortably.

GOLF SWING

Practice puts brains in your muscles.

~~~Sam Snead

The most common fault in golfers is to swing the club too hard or too fast. You lose control of the club head, lose your balance, and generally make poor contact with the ball. In other words, a swing that is too fast is not effective. The advice is always "slow it down."

The same advice applies to the performance of a repetition. In order to be most effective for your body, the rep must be slow, and the weight must be controlled through the entire range of motion. Often you see people performing reps of an exercise rapidly, and if you observe closely you determine that the reps are cheating reps, and not pure and honest. Momentum is moving the weight, and the target muscle is getting unwanted assistance from other muscle groups. Also, more than likely, too much weight is being used to be truly effective.

The best golf swing is a slow and smooth golf swing. The best rep is also a slow and controlled movement. The effectiveness of both a swing and a rep depends upon the proper mechanics and coordination of the movement. When you swing too hard or try to do a rep too fast your mechanics break down and the effectiveness is lost. A perfect golf swing adds value to the game because it creates a good result with the ball. A perfect rep adds value to the exercise by placing more stress on the muscle.

Why waste your time doing the least effective workout? Slow it down. If you are not lifting in perfect form, don't bother lifting at all. You are wasting your time.

TEMPO

Being deeply loved by someone gives you strength, while loving someone deeply gives you courage.

~~~Lao Tzo

My grandfather excelled at three sports that require proper tempo: golf, bowling, and pool. His delivery of the bowling ball, use of a pool cue, and his golf swing were smooth and at the same pace each time. I can recall many times that he advised me against rolling the bowling ball down the alley too hard. He would tell me to roll it smooth and easy to maintain proper control over the ball.

A repetition with a weight requires the same attention to tempo and pace. Smooth and easy does it. Do not rush it and always be under control.

ENJOYABLE TRAINING

The reward of a thing well done is to have done it.

~~~Ralph Waldo Emerson

Weight training is an enjoyable experience, both long and short term. In the long term, your efforts will be rewarded with improved health, appearance, and fitness. In the short term, each workout will be enjoyable if you learn to train safely for the congested feeling in the muscle, and recognize the feeling as an enjoyable product of the effort you have made. Imagine the wonder of the effort of an exercise literally going inside the muscle so that the tissue that you could not sense prior to the exercise is now pumped to the point of a sensual feeling.

To be successful in the pursuit of health and fitness in your training, you must train in a way that makes you feel good to do it. If you train in a way that causes you pain or makes you feel bad or depressed, you will soon give it up. The phrase "No pain-no gain" is ignorant and not a good thought to have while training. Pain does not indicate benefit. Pain hurts. Why do you want to do something that hurts? Think "no brain-no gain."

Train safely. Keep your weights and sets moderate to get a pump, perform pure reps, and maintain a positive and confident attitude toward exercise. Stupid training will rip up your body and affect your life. Train willingly and sensibly.

Confidence comes from knowing you will succeed by performing pure, precise reps, and not from trying to achieve a weight-rep goal. Don't think that each workout has to be a "hard workout." A "soft workout" is often just as productive, if not more so. Never leave the gym with the thought that you have failed. Recognize that your training time always has value.

Success in making lifestyle and health changes must come from a positive attitude based on doing something that makes you feel good. Avoid a negative attitude based upon guilt, i.e. that you have to exercise or diet because you have been guilty of laziness or overindulgence. Train because you want to do it, not because you think you have to do it.

Have a positive relationship with your training and enjoy it. Your relationship with your training should not create tension in your life by developing unnecessary anxiety and feelings of guilt. It is up to you to make your training enjoyable and seek the fulfillment that is the reason you train.

ADJUST YOUR TRAINING

If you don't like what you're doing, you can always pick up your needle and move to another groove.

~~~Timothy Leary

There will be times when your training will not create a pump that you can feel. The exercise is creating some congestion in the tissue, but for some reason you are unable to feel it. If you have trouble sensing a pump after a few sets, don't be concerned. The congestion is there, and the exercise has been productive for your health and well-being. There is no failure to the exercise merely because you cannot feel the pump. You just need to realize that it is not going to happen for you every time, but continue to have a pump that you can sense as one of your goals every workout.

Listen to the little voice within that tells you when it is time to decrease the poundage for a while to get the result you want to feel. You should recognize that many body factors like energy, fatigue, concentration, blood sugar level, and mental state vary on a daily basis. Therefore you should be flexible to adjust and reform your training according to your readiness to train.

Try to go to the gym with instinct and imagination. Be able to analyze what weight feels good that day and use it. Ask yourself what weight feels right to control to get the pure reps necessary to get a pump. Don't be afraid to change the exercise you are doing that day if it just does not feel comfortable. It is important to recognize this variation and adjust the workout to match the daily degree of change in those elements that affect your performance. When your "biorhythms" are down, train but lighten up on yourself. If the gym seems to be a burden and not a welcome diversion to your life, give yourself a break mentally and physically.

Training should be a respite from the hustle and bustle of your life. It's something you do for you, giving yourself the gift of good health.

VARIETY

Don't gamble on the future. Act now without delay.

~~~Simon de Beauvoir

One aspect of progressive resistance training which is often overlooked is the wide variety of available training techniques. When you make changes in your training, you place different types of stress on the body. This can lead to continued adaptation to the stress in the form of strength, development, conditioning, and improved appearance.

Some of the components of training you can vary are:

a. the amount of resistance you use for the movement;
b. the number of repetitions you do in a set (inversely proportionate to the amount of weight used);
c. the number of sets of an exercise;
d. the sequence of the exercises;
e. the number of exercises you choose to do per workout;
f. the amount of rest between sets and between exercises;
g. the rest time between training sessions;
h. the exercises chosen for each muscle group or individual muscle;
i. the placement of the hands on the bar or handle;
j. the placement of the feet while performing an exercise for the legs;
k. the pattern of resistance used while doing an exercise, i.e. increasing, decreasing, or maintaining the resistance from set to set;

l. training the entire body in one workout, or some body parts at one time, and other body parts at another time;

m. the type of equipment used, i.e. barbell, dumbbell, machines, pulleys, bodyweight.

Learn to be creative in your training by using the options available to constantly change the stress on your body and thereby force the muscles to continually adapt to new challenges. Keep the muscles confused with the stress you are creating to continue to improve your development.

PRE-EXHAUSTION

It does not matter how slowly you go as long as you do not stop.

~~~Confucius

A very good training method for creating muscle congestion quickly is known as pre-exhaustion. This is a training technique that can be used after a year or so of training.

When exercising just one muscle in a movement, and creating movement at just one joint, you are doing an isolation exercise. When exercising several muscles at one time, causing movement at more than one joint by the simultaneous contraction of separate muscles, you are doing a compound exercise for a muscle group.

Every individual muscle can function by itself to move a bone, or in conjunction with other muscles to move more than one bone. For example, the function of the triceps is to extend the forearm away from the upper arm. However, in combination with the deltoid muscle, the triceps enables you to extend your entire arm overhead. When doing a pressing exercise by pushing a bar overhead, you are using the deltoid to raise the upper arm bone and the triceps to straighten the arm at the elbow.

The problem is that a compound exercise involves muscles of different sizes and strengths. The primary muscle that is intended to be worked is usually the larger and stronger one. Working in combination, there is a "weak link" muscle that fatigues quicker than the other working muscles, typically due to size or leverage. When the weaker muscle tires and can no longer contract, the set ends before the larger muscle has been sufficiently worked.

The trick to the pre-exhaustion method is to minimize the effect of the weak link muscle by doing an isolation exercise for the larger muscle. You follow the isolation movement set immediately with a compound exercise set. The advantage to this type of training is how quickly you feel a sensation in the primary muscle. You are balancing the relative strength of the muscles by pre-exhausting the primary muscle so it is momentarily weaker than the smaller associated muscles.

For example, one of the basic compound movements for the shoulder muscles is the overhead press, using a barbell, dumbbells, or a machine. An isolation exercise for the deltoids is the dumbbell lateral raise (raising dumbbells with arms fairly straight to shoulder height to side or front). Do a set of lateral raises, 10-15 slow reps, and immediately do a set of overhead presses with a weight that will permit 10-15 pure reps. After a brief rest, repeat the cycle, and then focus your mind into your shoulder muscles to feel the effect of the exercise. There should be a significant feeling of congestion of blood in the deltoids. By pre-exhausting the larger deltoid muscle, you have maximized the benefit of the pressing exercise on the deltoids by minimizing the effect of the smaller triceps.

The same principle can be used for chest, back, and legs. Choose an isolation exercise for the larger muscle and a compound movement for the general area. Some examples are:

Chest

Isolation	Compound
Dumbbell flyes	Bench press
Machine flyes	Dips

Back

Isolation	Compound
Machine pullovers	Chins
Straight arm pulldowns	Lat pulldowns

Legs

Isolation	Compound
Leg extensions	Squats
Leg curls	Leg press

It is not necessary to do many pre-exhaustion sets to get a congested feeling in the muscle. Work until you feel the congestion, then stop. Do not be concerned with the amount of weight you are using in the compound movement. You will not be able to use as much resistance as you could if you did just the compound exercise alone, but the pump will be significantly greater. You should also change the exercises and use different combinations to keep the muscles confused.

Another form of the pre-exhaustion method is to do a few sets of an isolation exercise for the primary muscle, followed by sets of the compound exercise. This method is a bit less rigorous than the previously described super set method, and may be a better way to start into this type of program. Keep a good pace in this sequence by minimizing the rest between sets.

By using the pre-exhaustion method you are able to overcome the shortcomings of a compound exercise and make the exercise more effective. I have found this to be an excellent training method that saves time and accomplishes a quick pump in the muscle.

SUIT YOURSELF

Strength is not something you have, it's something you find.

~~~Emma Smith

One of the great benefits of any exercise program is that it can be designed to meet individual needs. As I stated previously, not all of the suggestions in this book are suitable for everyone. I have mentioned a general idea that doing compound exercises is a good training strategy. However, if your goal is to train for general fitness, there is nothing wrong with doing isolation exercises for a muscle.

For example, leg extensions and leg curls are more than adequate to develop and strengthen the legs. Squats may not be your best exercise for this purpose, and if you force yourself to do them, you may get frustrated or injure yourself. Do not think that a compound movement is absolutely necessary for your own personal beneficial training.

Some examples of isolation exercises:

Chest:
Dumbbell flyes
Machine flyes

Shoulders:
Dumbbell lateral raises
Cable lateral raises

Legs:
Leg extensions
Leg curls
Calf raises

Back:
Dumbbell pullovers on bench
Straight arm pulldowns on lat machine

Biceps:
Various curl movements

Triceps:
Cable pressdowns
Overhead extensions

Always remember that you must learn to do the exercise correctly and focus on pure rep performance. Train safely, no matter what type of exercise you do.

ABDOMINAL MUSCLES

People do not lack strength; they lack will.

~~~Victor Hugo

The muscles that protect the internal organs in the abdominal cavity are known, appropriately enough, as the abdominal muscles, or "abs." When developed and visible, this muscle group indicates fitness; generally the abdominal muscles are not prominent and visible unless there is an absence of body fat.

Body fat tends to accumulate in the abdominal area, and as a result this body part has been subject to much misinformation. The concept that performing hundreds of reps of situps or leg raises will burn off the fat and develop the muscle has been around for a long time. Good luck if you have the time and want to experiment with the theory.

Your dietary habits will determine the accumulation or the loss of fat in the area. Increased cardiovascular exercise will also enhance the loss of fat tissue. You cannot spot reduce one part of the body. If you want to lose weight from the abdominal area, you must lose weight from the entire body by ingesting fewer calories than you use.

As far as development of the protective muscle tissue, the abdominal muscles are like any other muscle group. They have a specific function; i.e. pulling one part of the skeleton toward another part. In this case, the sternum is pulled closer to the pelvis. The abdominal muscles respond to exercise in the same manner as other muscles. Sets of 10-20 reps, properly done, will develop the muscle.

Abdominal crunches, leg raises of various types, hanging leg raises, and other movements involving the abs should be done slowly, smoothly, and in good form. Stop the movement while in the fully contracted position before extending to the starting point. Start each rep slowly so that your abdominal muscles are controlling the movement, and not momentum.

For crunches, think of your upper body as the end of a carpet rolling up and then unrolling. Use your muscles to roll your upper body into a ball.

One key to abdominal exercises is constant tension to create a cramping and burning sensation in the tissue. When done properly, it will not take many reps to get this feeling. Twenty reps done correctly is better than 100 done incorrectly.

PYRAMID

We gain the strength of the temptation we resist.

~~~Ralph Waldo Emerson

The pyramid pattern of doing sets of an exercise has progressively increasing weight with the first few sets and decreasing weight with the final sets. Begin with a light weight as a warm-up set for 15-20 reps, and gradually increase the weight up to a set of 8-12 reps. Then decrease the weight on the final sets, again keeping the reps in the 8-12 range.

Here is an example of a pyramid workout:

135 lbs. x 12 reps

155 lbs. x 12 reps

185 lbs. x 8-12 reps

155 lbs. x 8-12 reps

135 lbs. x 8-12 reps

Keep your rest time between sets to a minimum to enhance your pump. Resist the temptation to do a maximum weight set for low reps at the top of the pyramid. You are training, not testing or demonstrating your strength.

Think in terms of the resistance being heavy for the number of reps you are doing in the top set. The resistance becomes a challenge at the twelfth rep so as to require a greater effort.

CARDIO

The secret of getting ahead is getting started.

~~~Mark Twain

Your conditioning program should always include a form of cardiovascular exercise. One cannot deny the positive effects of exercise that increases your heart rate over an extended period of time.

In the same way that you should recognize the variables available in weight training, you should also use a variety of exercises for cardiovascular training. Low impact exercises like bike riding may be best in the long run, and you should be conscious of the stress that some exercises, like running, place on body joints.

Experiment with doing your cardio work on the same day you do your resistance training or on different days. If your goal is to decrease your bodyweight, emphasize cardiovascular exercise over weight training. You will burn up more calories and enhance the prospect of losing weight. Patiently coax your cardiovascular conditioning for gradual long-term improvement.

My training in this area includes the treadmill and elliptical equipment. I create variety in these exercises by changing performance in creative ways. Sometimes I do a non-stop time on both machines. Other times I create a "superset" and do a couple of alternate sets of lesser time. For example, one day I might do 30 straight minutes on the elliptical and 30 minutes on the treadmill. Another day, I might alternate 15 minute "sets" i.e. 15 minutes on the elliptical, then 15 minutes on the treadmill, and so forth. In other words, I play with the time to make it less boring.

Fitness can be equated to how well the circulatory system delivers oxygen and nutrients to the tissues of the body. The more efficiently this delivery system works, the more fit and healthy you will become. Organic efficiency, which is the proper functioning of the glands and organs and the proper assimilation of food and drink, is the cornerstone of good health.

DON'T DO SINGLES

The cautious seldom err.

~~~Confucius

Training with the goal to improve health and appearance is not the same as testing your strength. Anyone can simply lie on a bench and attempt a single limit repetition in the bench press. However, this is not the equivalent of training, and it will do little if anything to improve health and appearance.

Testing your strength is the avoidance of the work necessary to improve your fitness. True training requires the effort and mental discipline to consistently work hard and do the sets and reps necessary to create congestion in the muscle tissue. Exercise your muscles, not your ego.

Weight training is not weightlifting. One of the longstanding problems with training has been the incorrect correlation with competitive weightlifting. The connection has created a bogus emphasis on the use of weight that is too heavy to be safe and effective. Resistance training is exercise, not weightlifting to test strength.

An increase in strength is the improved ability to control a weight for a number of reps in a rep scheme. An increase can occur for one rep or for 10 reps. In either event, strength has improved. If you increase your ability to bench press 185 pounds from 10 reps to 15 reps, you have increased your strength for that poundage. If you increase your ability to lift a poundage for 10 reps from 185 pounds to 225 pounds, you have also increased your strength.

Therefore, do not think of strength increase as only for a single repetition.

**Don't lift the weight,
Exercise the muscle.**

TENDONS AND LIGAMENTS

If you refuse to accept anything but the best, you very often get it.

~~~W. Somerset Maugham

The tissue that connects a bone to another bone is a ligament. The tissue that connects a muscle to a bone is a tendon. Both tendons and ligaments are of necessity strong tissues, but each is subject to injuries which can often be permanent or require surgery.

You risk damage to these connective tissues by using excessive weight and/or training with bad form. An injury can occur immediately or develop over time. Remember this: the true risk to stupid training is damage to your tendons and ligaments. Once injured, the tissue is never the same and will cause you eternal pain.

One advantage to training for a congested feeling is that you are not placing as much stress on the connective tissue. By using moderate weight for higher repetitions in perfect form, the stress is focused for the most part on the muscle tissue. Train to exercise the muscle, not to damage the connective tissue.

Take good care of the tendons and ligaments in your body. You are going to need the use of them for your entire life. Train sensibly in good form and in moderation to avoid injury to these tissues.

CHANGE THE WORKOUT

You have the power over your mind—not outside events.
Realize this and you will find strength.

~~~Marcus Aurelius

Do not be afraid to change either the exercise you are using or the manner in which you use the exercise. You do not want your body – or your mind – to get bored. Stay outside of a boxed training method.

There are several ways to create variety in your workouts. One is to change the exercises done for a body part. Another is to change the performance of the exercise. As an example, some variations of performance of the bench press are:

1. Straight sets (consecutive sets with the same weight);
2. Pyramid sets (increase weight for a few sets, then decrease the weight for the final sets);
3. Extended sets (decrease the weight at the end of the set and continue the exercise without stopping, then decrease the weight again and continue without stopping);
4. Pre-exhaustion (isolation movement for the chest muscles done prior to the bench press);
5. Super set (do a set of bench presses immediately followed by an exercise for another body part, e.g. chins for the back);
6. 10 x 10 (do ten sets of ten reps with only 60 seconds of rest between sets - adjust the weight to permit ten reps as the sets progress);

7. Change the exercise in the same day (i.e. do some straight sets followed by an extended set).

This list is not intended to be exhaustive. In fact, the variety you create is limited only by your imagination. The constant theme should always be doing perfect reps and the most work in the least time.

SUPERSET

What is to give light must endure burning.

~~~Anton Wildgaus

One popular training method is known as a superset. It is a broad term that generally refers to the performance of one set of an exercise immediately followed by a set of a different exercise. The pre-exhaustion routine is one form of a superset that targets a specific muscle by working it with a set of an isolation exercise followed by a compound exercise that works the target muscle. For example, a pre-exhaustion superset for the shoulders might include a set of dumbbell lateral raises followed by a set of barbell overhead presses.

Another combination of exercises for a superset focuses on the antagonistic muscle groups of the body. One exercise moves the bones in one direction, and the other moves the bones in the opposite direction; thus, the term antagonistic.

An antagonistic superset for the arms would include a biceps exercise and a triceps exercise. One might perform a set of a curling exercise using the biceps, immediately followed by a set of pushdowns on the lat machine for triceps. One muscle is pulling the forearm toward the upper arm, and the other is extending the forearm away from the upper arm. After a short rest, the sequence is repeated. The feeling of congestion is enhanced because it is focused on the adjoining muscles. One theory has it that while one muscle is working, the other muscle recovers more quickly from the set just completed.

Analyze your body structure to determine other possible combinations for supersets. I think it best to try to keep the congestion and feeling in the same general area of the body by working muscles that complement each other. For example, a push-pull superset, doing a chest exercise followed by a back exercise, keeps blood flow in the upper body. Experiment for yourself to see what combinations give you results.

THE BASICS

Good habits formed at youth make all the difference.

~~~Aristotle

You have to know and develop the perfect performance of an exercise.

You must know the correct and effective application of the exercise movement to the muscle.

You must develop an accurate calculation of the amount of work that is appropriate for your individual ability to recuperate from the exercise effort.

SQUATS

Somebody should tell us, right at the start of our lives, that we are dying. Then we might live life to the limit, every minute of every day. Do it! I say. Whatever you want to do, do it now! There are only so many tomorrows.

~~~Pope Paul VI

Squats are the best total body exercise. Hard work on this movement over time will yield tremendous results.

Keep the reps in each set fairly high. Ten to twenty is a good range. Use a moderate weight and get good advice on the proper form. Always keep the back flat, chest out, and look at a spot that is eye level during the set. Never bounce from the bottom. Stay under control during the entire repetition. Do not go below a point where the top of the thigh is parallel to the ground. You should avoid a strong lock-out of the knees at the top of the rep. In fact, try to keep moving, like a well-oiled piston.

Do a couple of sets of leg extensions, leg curls, and hyperextensions prior to your sets of squats. These movements will warm up the knees and lower back, which are the hinging parts of the body that are affected by the squat movement.

Respect the squat exercise for what it can do for you, but also for the potential for injury if done improperly. This exercise has several large muscle groups working in unison to do the movement. The result is that it builds the nervous system in a way that affects the entire body. Remember, however, that squats may not be safe for your body due to prior injuries or your body structure.

A NUMBER DOES NOT
MAKE A GOOD WORKOUT

The greatest of follies is to sacrifice health for any other kind of happiness.

~~~Arthur Schopenhauer

A common fault in training is to try to develop a qualitative analysis of the time spent training by subjecting the time and effort to a quantitative analysis. In other words, there may be a tendency to equate the quality of an exercise session with the numbers that attach to the effort. Amount of weight, number of reps with a certain weight, and number of sets are all components of a good and enjoyable workout to some people.

This is the wrong attitude to have in your training. It creates an internal pressure to make the training effort equate to an arbitrary number, and thus some thought of success or failure attaches to the number and to the perceived quality of the training session. Do not have a weight-rep goal. You are setting yourself up for disappointment and frustration.

You should avoid this habit. In the short term, perform pure reps and create the pumped feeling as your goals. Over a period of time, the "numbers" (amount of resistance, number of reps) that are part of your exercise choices will increase. Don't make the number your goal. Instead, focus on the quality of each repetition and creating a feeling in the muscle. The numbers it takes to reach this goal are not important. Each workout presents a challenge that should not be a number.

Do you really think that you should enjoy a workout more based on a number associated with an exercise poundage or repetitions? Should you like your training if you did 10 reps with a weight but dislike your training if you only did 8 reps? Come on. Why would you ever want to make training a negative experience?

There was a time in my training when I could do 11 reps on the dip bars with 130 pounds tied to me at a bodyweight of 170 pounds. My incorrect focus at that time was on the numbers rather than the quality of training. I recall that a workout would become a success/failure experience: successful if I did 11 reps, and failure if I did not do 11 reps. Rather than a workout being a consistently pleasant experience, I dealt with a positive/negative situation created by a bogus weight-rep goal. I should have realized that on some days I would be stronger than other days, and adjusted the resistance and workout accordingly. Instead I let my ego interfere with the quality of my training.

Strive to eliminate the negative by avoiding the quantity and focusing on the quality. Stay positive and be patient. Develop an instinct for the range of reps you have done in a set and the weight and range that are needed to create a feeling in the muscle. Avoid the distraction and possible frustration of numbers.

DON'T DO A ROUTINE

Beloved, I pray that all may go well with you and that you may be in good health, just as it is well with your soul.

~~~3 John 1:2

The term "training routine" has been used to define a group of exercises that are done consistently over time. People often think there is an absolute exercise that suits them for a particular muscle group, and if they find and stick with it forever, guaranteed success will follow.

The body adapts to an exercise movement done a specific way. Thus, the concept of a routine is not beneficial for effective exercise. Do not think in terms of doing the same exercises the same way over a long period of time. Do not feed your ego from the ability to do a certain movement with a certain weight. Instead, recognize that changing training techniques will require your muscles to consistently adapt to different stress. The only routine you should use is one of continued and consistent safe training of all the muscle groups in the body.

Above all, do not be afraid to change the exercises you are using or the performance of the exercises. It may be easier to follow a packaged method of training than to risk experimenting and changing to determine what is right for your body at a particular time – but the packaged method will be far less effective.

Learn the different exercise movements available for the muscle groups. With the variety of equipment available to work the same general exercise, it is easy to change the stress. For example, the bench press can be performed in the traditional manner on a bench with a barbell, but there is equipment made to imitate the movement in a variety of ways. Use everything available for this purpose. You will be able to create new arrangements of exercises, avoid becoming stale, and enhance your development. Avoid the training routine.

SPORTS, STRENGTH, AND ENDURANCE

If you are distressed by anything external, the pain is not due to the thing itself, but your estimate of it; and this you have the power to revoke at any moment.

~~~Marcus Antonius

If you are training to improve your performance in an athletic activity, choose a resistance that forces you to make a strong effort in the 10-15 repetition range. The goal is to train for both strength and endurance. The effort on the last rep forces your mind to recruit the maximum number of muscle fibers at a time when the tissue is fatigued. In most sports, you need a combination and balance between strength and endurance. Also, forcing yourself to do this rep range develops the mental discipline to fight through fatigue with continued effort.

I trained at a gym with a fellow who was an All-American football player at the time. He never did fewer than 10 reps per set on his exercises. When asked the inevitable, "How much can you lift?" question, his reply was that he did not know because he never did maximum weight sets to test his strength. His reasoning was simple. His method of training was designed to make him as strong in the fourth quarter as he was in the first quarter. You cannot achieve this result by testing yourself with heavy weights and low reps.

HEAVY-LIGHT

Do not pray for easy lives. Pray to be stronger men.

~~~John F. Kennedy

The opposite of pre-exhaustion is the heavy-light system. Perform a compound movement for a particular group, followed by an isolation exercise for the primary muscle. Complete the sets of the compound movement and follow with sets of the isolation movement.

For example, for the chest you might do a few sets of the bench press, followed by a few sets of flyes with dumbbells or on a machine. Keep the rep range for the compound movement between 8-12, but do a higher number of reps for the isolation exercise. Minimize the rest time between sets. Focus on a target muscle with the isolation movement and create a feeling of blood congestion in the tissue.

This training method is a basic and sound way to combine the benefits of a compound exercise with an isolation exercise. Be creative and use it for shoulders, legs and back as well.

BODY CONTACT

Happiness is that state of consciousness which proceeds from the achievement of one's values.

~~~Ayn Rand

In any exercise, think about the part of the skeleton that is moving in the exercise, as opposed to counting reps or thinking success/failure about the set. Get your mind to think about the movement involved.

For example, nearly all upper body exercises involve the movement of the arms and hands in some manner. Try focusing on the hands, and the movement of the hand through each repetition. Since the hand is the only part of your body that is in contact with the bar, it is easier to sense both the movement of the hand and the resistance being moved. This combination creates a better mental connection to the muscle or muscles being worked. Be patient with this concept, and it will improve your ability to feel the effect of the exercise at the end of the set.

PUSH –PULL

Short as life is, we make it still shorter by the careless waste of time.

~~~Victor Hugo

A good combination of exercises for the upper body is based on the movement of the bones in the arms. The arms can push something away from you, or pull something toward you. The pushing movement involves the chest/shoulder muscle groups, and the pulling movement involves the back muscle group. Because these are adjoining muscle groups, it is a good idea to work them in the same workout or in sequence to keep blood flow to the same area of the body.

You can start by doing a straight set sequence, i.e. do your chest exercises followed by your back exercises. After you have been training for a year or so, try a superset of a compound pushing exercise with a compound pulling exercise. Perform a set of a chest exercise immediately followed by a set of a back exercise. The sequence of chest-back or back-chest is arbitrary, but the combination will cause increased blood flow to the same general section of the body, and hence greater congestion in a shorter time. Some examples of the exercises are:

PUSH

Dips
Bench Press

PULL

Lat machine pulldowns
Chins
Seated pulley rowing

A typical superset sequence might be dips-chins, bench press-pulldowns, or any combination that you prefer. Keep the rest between the two exercise sets to a minimum. For example, do a set of dips and immediately do a set of chins. Rest a couple of minutes, and then repeat the sequence. Keep the number of reps high. Do 3-5 sets and you will feel the congestion in both the chest muscles and the back muscles.

EXTENDED SET

Gladness of the heart is the life of a man, and the joyfulness of a man prolongs his days.

~~~Ecclesiasticus 30:22

Another excellent method of creating muscle congestion quickly is an extended or multi-poundage set. After a couple of warm-up sets of an exercise, pick a weight that you know by experience will permit 8-12 reps in good form. Do a set of pure reps, then decrease the resistance significantly and immediately do another set. Do not count reps, but have in mind that you are doing 8-12 in the set. When the second set is completed, decrease the weight again and immediately do another set of 8-12 reps. If you are up to it, do a fourth set with less weight.

This method lets you extend the set by decreasing the weight when you have reached a fatigue point in the muscle. The weight for each set feels as heavy as the weight used for the previous sets. If necessary, repeat the cycle until you feel the congestion of blood in the muscle tissue.

I have found this method to be extremely effective for getting a pump in the muscle. It is particularly suited to exercise equipment that has a weight stack with a pin or other device to easily change the weight.

DIPS

Bar dips is the premier exercise for the muscles of the upper body that push and extend the arms away from the torso (pectorals, deltoids and triceps). Dips are for the upper body what squats are for the lower part of your body.

I first wrote about this exercise in Iron Man magazine several years ago. When I was training competitively, dips was by far my primary upper body exercise. I rarely did the bench press because of the great results I achieved from dips. When I coached, I also emphasized this exercise for the athletes with whom I worked. I recall that I could do very few reps when I first started doing the exercise. Eventually I was able to use 130 pounds tied to me for sets of 11 reps, and my upper body development increased as well.

If possible, use a dip apparatus that has bars which are not parallel, so as to accommodate various body widths. Use a steady and controlled technique. Keep your chin on your chest, bend your legs, and cross your ankles. Lower yourself by bending your arms so your body descends to a point at which you feel comfortable; pause, and then push yourself up to the starting position. Do not go lower than a point where your upper arms are parallel with the floor. Do your reps smoothly with no jerky movements. One reason this exercise is so beneficial is because it is hard to cheat on the movement.

Most people find the exercise difficult and uncomfortable initially. If you cannot push yourself up from the bottom position, simply start at the top position and lower yourself slowly to the bottom. Get off the bars, stand up, and resume the starting position at the top with your arms straight and repeat the "lowering" phase. Some gyms have machines that assist you in doing the movement until you can do it on your own.

Give your body time to adapt and to develop the coordination needed to do the exercise correctly. Gradually increase to sets of 15 reps. When 15 reps becomes easy, consider using weight for additional resistance. You can use a machine made for the exercise, or a belt with a chain made to add weight by running the chain through the holes in the plates.

Work this exercise hard for a while as your only upper body exercise for the pushing muscles. You will witness a significant improvement in your chest, shoulders, and arms.

DUMBBELLS

Every man is the builder of a temple called his body.

~~~Henry David Thoreau

One of the best ways to create variety in your training is to use dumbbells in an exercise movement. Nearly every exercise that can be done with both arms can also be done with each individual arm.

The use of dumbbells requires more coordination and control of the muscle. Dumbbell training creates a unique stress on the muscles and nervous system. You must concentrate more on the effort when using a dumbbell. This focus can increase the safety of the exercise. Given enough time and practice, the use of dumbbells will improve your strength, conditioning and appearance.

CHEST SPRING EXPANDERS

When your values are clear to you, making decisions becomes easier.

~~~Roy E. Disney

A form of exercise equipment that has been around for many years is known as a chest spring expander. It has two handles that are connected by springs, bands or cables that stretch and can be adjusted in number to create more or less resistance. In the same way you can add weight to a bar to increase the resistance in a barbell exercise, you can add another cable, spring or band over time to increase the resistance with this equipment.

A major advantage that the expander has over barbells is the resistance increases when the handles are pulled farther apart as the tension in the cables increases. A standard weight exercise has a constant tension from the pull of gravity.

There are several exercises that can be done with this equipment. I have found it effective for the curling movement for the arms. Place a foot in one handle on the floor and slowly pull the other handle by bending one arm with the elbow at the side. Resist the pull of the spring as the arm straightens. For triceps, stabilize one handle overhead in some fashion and do a pressdown movement. You can research other exercise movements as well.

No matter what exercise you are doing, you are still working with the pull of the spring as the resistance in both parts of the movement. Use this equipment for variety in your exercise program.

THE GOAL

Exercise to stimulate, not to annihilate. The world wasn't formed in a day and neither were we. Set small goals and build on them.

~~~Lee Haney
8x Mr. Olympia

Your training session is not an ego trip. It has a specific goal, and that goal has nothing to do with creating an impression on any other person. The goal is to perform pure reps to create a congested feeling in the muscle that you can sense as the effect of the exercise.

To emphasize the need to get a sensory connection or feeling between the brain and the muscle being worked, I suggest you wear loose clothing that essentially covers most of your body. You do not have to see yourself in order to create a feeling in the muscle tissue. If anything, the visual image may be more of a distraction to your focus on the repetition. It is more productive to avoid the visual awareness that occurs if you are wearing just shorts and a tank top. Wear something that covers most of your body and forces you to sense the muscle without being able to see it. It is better to feel it than to see it.

OVERTRAINING

You never know what is enough until you know what is more than enough.

~~~William Blake

Exercise is stress, and the body adapts by changing to increase its ability to deal with the stress the next time it occurs. However, too much stress has a negative effect on the mind and body. If you are going to make a mistake, make it on the side of doing too little training rather than too much. The basic framework of your training program must be based on the principle of stress followed by rest and recovery.

Overtraining taxes your body's recuperation ability and poses a risk of injury to your muscles, tendons and ligaments. Further, overtraining makes it much more difficult to create congestion in the muscle tissue, and makes you mentally stale. There is a limit to the amount of exercise that benefits your body. Anything more than what you can handle is abusive and not healthy work.

It is impossible to create one rule that applies to everyone regarding exercise frequency because we each have our own individual tolerance for exercise. The fact is that you must give a muscle sufficient time to recuperate between training sessions. The choice depends on your sense of whether the muscle has properly recovered from the last workout, and also the time available for training. One option is to give yourself two or three days of rest between workouts for a muscle group. This schedule can be done in total body workouts or split body workouts. A couple of days should provide sufficient rest and leave you physically and mentally ready to benefit from the next workout.

You really must develop the ability to sense when you are too fatigued to train because your mind and muscles have not properly recovered from the last workout. Listen to your body when it tells you to lighten up or lay off a workout. If you feel "hung over" from your training, you have abused your body and need rest. Obey your body. Of course, you also must distinguish between needing rest and being a bit lazy.

Overtraining also occurs when too much is done in one workout. Too many sets and too many exercises can create too much stress. A large volume of exercise is not good.

Training hard is not the same as training a long time. Work hard and safely to create congestion in the muscle, and then stop. Any more work done beyond the point of congestion is counter-productive. The body will not recover adequately when you overtrain and you will get frustrated. Again, err on the side of too little rather than too much.

Determine a workout for the maximum pump with the minimum number of sets. Do not be excessive in your training. The person who makes the quickest gains is the one who knows when to stop.

When people fail in their efforts to make exercise a regular part of their lifestyle, it is rarely because they did not train hard enough. Instead, failure usually occurs because a person works too hard and finds it unpleasant or gets injured.

HYPERTROPHY

Tell him to live by yes and no—yes to everything good, no to everything bad.

~~~William James

Muscle growth is called hypertrophy. A decrease in muscle size is called atrophy. Muscle tissue atrophies significantly due to lack of use when a leg is in a cast. Once the cast is removed, hypertrophy occurs as the muscle grows in response to increased use.

One interesting phenomenon is called muscle memory. When you first begin training, it takes time for muscle growth to occur. Over time, you experience an increase in size and shape of the muscle tissue. If you quit training, a bit of atrophy occurs due to the lack of accustomed use. However, if you resume training, the muscle will regain its former size quicker than was required the first time. The body "remembers" the motor pathways and coordination that it developed the first time, thus making strength and growth easier. Think of it as a balloon that is difficult to inflate the first time, but easier to inflate a second time.

Keep this idea in mind if you have to stop training for a while, but then resume. You can expect to experience muscle hypertrophy faster once you resume than you did when you first started.

TOTAL BODY WORKOUT

A long habit of not thinking a thing wrong gives it a superficial appearance of being right.

~~~Thomas Paine

If you are training to improve your performance in a sport, train all the major muscle groups so as to have balanced strength and coordination throughout the entire body. If your sport requires the consistent movement of a particular part of the skeleton, focus some extra effort on the muscle groups that produce that movement. Do not train just the muscle that is sport-specific. Balanced development and strength is necessary for long term success. Also, you will be using your entire body for your lifetime, long after you cease playing a sport. For athletics and for the long term, it makes sense to stay focused on total body development.

Don't sacrifice one muscle group for another. True strength and fitness comes from properly training all muscle groups. They support each other.

Your goal should be to gain strength in your entire body safely, efficiently, effectively, and with a patient attitude. Once you have created this foundation, work to apply the strength to your given sport.

ANTAGONISTIC MUSCLES

The man who knows right from wrong and has good judgment and common sense is happier than the man who is immensely rich.

~~~Proverbs

You should work for balanced development and strength in the antagonistic muscles, i.e. muscles that move bones in the opposite direction. Your appearance will suffer if one muscle is much stronger than the opposite muscle. I also believe that you risk injury if you exercise a muscle that moves a bone in one direction to the exclusion of the other muscle, such that you have an imbalance in relative strength.

For example, I have seen athletes train the quadriceps (frontal thigh muscles), and neglect the hamstrings (muscles at the back of upper leg). The result is an imbalance in strength, and oftentimes leads to injury to the weaker hamstring muscles when running.

For better appearance and to avoid injury, give equal attention to the antagonistic muscles.

BALANCED LEG DEVELOPMENT

The obvious is that which is never seen until someone expresses it simply.

~~~Khalil Gibran

If you are interested in improving your running speed, concentrate on your hamstring strength at least as much as quadriceps development. Check out the back of the thighs on the best sprinters and you will see a mass of muscle as large as the quadriceps in the front. In addition, working the hamstrings adds to stability in the knee joint.

A good sequence I have used is to alternate the leg extension for the front quadriceps with the leg curl movement for the rear hamstrings. Keep the reps in the 12-20 range. Hold each rep in the fully contracted position for a couple of seconds. Do a full, slow, and smooth movement through the entire range of motion. Add in an extended set on occasion. Vary the placement of your feet and flex the muscles between sets. Train for a congested feeling in the muscle.

WEAK LINK

It is a man's own mind, not his enemy or foe, that leads him to evil ways.

~~~Buddha

A compound exercise requires the simultaneous coordination and integration of several separate muscles to move bones against resistance. Compound movements are the basic exercises, i.e. bench press, overhead press, chins, squats, etc. Note, however, that within any compound exercise some muscles are larger than others involved in the movement. The smaller muscles are the "weak links" in the chain and will fatigue prior to the larger muscle.

Analyze the exercise and determine the major muscle and the associated smaller, weak links. Common sense would tell you not to exercise one of the smaller muscles prior to performing the compound movement. For example, training your triceps prior to doing the bench press movement will restrict the effect on the chest muscles, because the smaller triceps has been fatigued. Do not work the "weak link" muscle with an isolation movement prior to doing the compound exercise.

CONCENTRATION

It is easier to build strong children than to repair broken men.

~~~Frederick Douglass

Creating the proper focus and concentration while performing an exercise movement is important to obtain the most benefit. There is no accepted, tried and true method to create the maximum concentration. One often reads that the mind has to get into the muscle, i.e., a sensory feeling in the target muscle while doing the exercise. Generally, this is difficult to do, and it detracts from the concentration on the movement itself to do a perfect rep.

Depending on the exercise, one method I have found beneficial is to focus on the hand or foot as it is moving through a plane of motion. The hand or foot is typically the only part of your body in contact with the equipment, so it is easy to sense it during the movement. Also, think about the normal movement of the hand or foot as if you are doing something else. If you are doing a curling movement, focus on the hand moving toward your face. Try to ignore the resistance and simply focus on the effort to pull your hand to your face.

Taking it a step further, imagine you are doing something that ultimately requires a fine detail movement by the hand. For example, when you brush your teeth, the movement of the hand toward the head becomes more focused and "fine tuned" as the hand approaches the mouth and places the brush on the small area of the teeth. Put this type of focus into the curling movement, or any other movement. Imagine that you are using the muscles to perform an ordinary task, as the muscle is designed to function. You have to focus on the hand for most upper body movements and the feet for lower body movements. Put a glass in a cupboard using pressing movements. Kick a ball doing leg extensions. Reach for something while working triceps.

Ultimately, if you concentrate on either your hand or your foot as you would when performing an ordinary task you will do the repetition slower and under greater control. This focus will translate into better muscle control against the resistance you are using because you are consciously using the motor pathway between your brain and the muscle to control the movement. Think about moving your hand or foot slowly each repetition.

THE BRACHIALIS MUSCLE

There is little that can withstand a man who can conquer himself.
　　~~~Louis XIV

If you want a larger, stronger, and more toned muscle to flex the forearm up to the upper arm, work the brachialis muscle prior to exercising the biceps. The brachialis lies under the biceps, and is also a flexor responsible for bending the arm. Do an exercise to congest the brachialis before exercising the biceps. If you congest the biceps first, the muscle tissue presses down into the brachialis and makes it more difficult to properly work that muscle.

To pump the brachialis, do reverse curls (a curl movement with the palms down instead of up) and hammer curls (dumbbell curls with the thumb turned upwards, like you are using a hammer). Do your reps slowly and in perfect form.

THE TRICEPS

Great works are performed not by strength but by perseverance.

~~~Samuel Johnson

The triceps muscle extends the forearm away from the upper arm, i.e. straightens the arm. This muscle is much larger than the flexors of the arm (biceps, brachialis). Well-developed triceps create more impressive upper arm development. Also, working the triceps keeps the muscle toned and helps avoid the flabbiness that can develop in the back of the arm.

The triceps get indirect stimulation in compound exercises like the bench press, dips, and the overhead press. Work an isolation exercise for the triceps like triceps pressdowns after the compound movement for direct work on the muscle.

REP RANGE AND TIME

No man is hurt but by himself.

~~~Diogenes

Choose an exercise poundage that permits you to do 8-12 pure reps. Use enough weight in perfect form to make the last rep fairly difficult to complete but not the absolute last rep you can do in the set. This range of repetitions will increase blood flow to the muscles being worked, thus creating a feeling of congestion.

Keep your rest time between sets to a minimum. A minute or two should be your goal, but develop your own sense of the correct time for you. Maintain a fast pace by minimizing the rest. The quicker the pace the more athletic the workout.

Have you ever noticed the difference in the physiques of a sprinter and a long distance runner? Both may do the same amount of work, but the sprinter does it in much less time, and thus has better muscular development.

Do not wander far from the equipment you are using. Do a set, maybe discreetly flex the muscle you trained to get a feeling in it, and then do the next set after a minute or two. Adjust the poundage if necessary to maintain the range of repetitions. Always try to do the most work in the least possible time for the most benefit in your training. I usually count to 60 or thereabouts between sets in order to keep the pace I want to maintain.

Remember that the amount of weight that you use for an exercise does not matter nearly as much as the quality of work and effort your muscles are forced to do, the time in which you do the work, and the safety of your set.

Learn the application of specific exercises to general muscle function and skeletal movement. Recognize that all exercise movements are built around the skeletal movements of the arms, legs, and torso. Think of an exercise as simply a muscle moving a bone in its natural plane of motion, against some form of resistance.

TEN SETS OF TEN

We are what we repeatedly do. Excellence, then, is not an act but a habit.

~~~Aristotle

As with all good advice, there is bound to be an exception. Throughout this book, I stress that numbers are not relevant to a good workout and generally discourage you from counting reps in your set. Well, I will now make a slight exception to that general rule, and call it ten sets of ten.

This method will create a great pump in a short period of time. You are going to do ten sets of ten reps of only one exercise per muscle group per workout. Do a set of ten reps, wait a minute or two, and do another set of ten reps. Repeat this pattern until you have done ten sets with little rest between sets. You will have to decrease the poundage as you do the sets but do not worry about the weight. You will feel a pump as you progress through the sets, no matter the amount of resistance. The amount of weight is of secondary concern.

Begin this training technique with fewer than ten sets, according to your own comfort level. Also, you might take a full two minutes or so between sets. Try to increase to ten sets and decrease the time to 60 seconds.

This technique is a great example of doing the most work in the least possible time. Try it on a body part for a few workouts to force it to adapt to a new stress. Do just one exercise for the muscle group in that workout. For example, if you are training your chest, do just the bench press in your workout and do ten sets of ten. Do not do another chest exercise in that workout session.

This technique will improve blood circulation to the muscle group and will also improve the neuromuscular control you have in the exercise. I recommend that you have a year or so of training experience before you do this training method.

SPECIFIC EXERCISES

Everybody, sooner or later, sits down to a banquet of consequences.

~~~R.L. Stevenson

Here is some advice for specific exercises. Most of these points apply to standard barbell and dumbbell equipment and machines that duplicate the standard movements.

BENCH PRESS

1. Try not to lie flat on the bench. Press your shoulder blades together when you lie against the bench and keep that posture throughout the set. This position will make a shorter distance to push the bar and will decrease the risk of injury by forcing you to stay in one position as the set progresses.

2. Plant your feet firmly on the floor, with the knee bent at slightly less than 90 degrees. Push the foot into the floor when doing the exercise to stabilize the body.

3. As you slowly lower the bar, let the elbows bend away from the body. Pause at the chest for a full second, without relaxing, so that you are pushing from a dead stop. Push the bar up smoothly and slowly. Don't arch your back or your hips. Avoid forcefully straightening the arms by keeping the elbows bent slightly at the top. Pause briefly at the top. Think of your arms as a pneumatic piston, moving smoothly and under control.

4. Use a shoulder width grip. Wide hand spacing hurts your shoulders. You want to evenly distribute the resistance throughout the entire upper body without undue stress on any one muscle or the shoulder joint.

5. Lower the bar slowly to the same point on the chest for each rep. You should determine the spot from which you can push with the best leverage and strength. Press the bar up and back toward your head.

6. Do not turn this exercise into a trampoline bounce off of the chest. Use the upper body muscles to push the weight from a dead stop on the chest.

CHIN UPS/LAT MACHINE PULLDOWNS.

1. Start each rep with the arms fully extended. Pull smoothly and extend your arms back to the starting position in a controlled manner.

2. As you pull the bar closer to your torso, arch the back so that you can pull the bar to your chest. Try to squeeze the shoulder blades together. Pause when the bar is at the chest. Do the reps smoothly and slowly.

3. Vary the grip and the hand spacing, but don't go much beyond shoulder width.

4. If you are doing chin ups, the weight of your body is the resistance, and you cannot vary it as you can with lat machine pulldowns. You may not be able to do many reps at first. Don't let this prevent you from staying with the

exercise. Get some assistance in the form of a partner standing behind you lifting up on your feet to help you pull yourself up, then slowly lower yourself down to the starting position. Be persistent and let your body adapt to the movement.

BICEPS CURLS

1. Start with arms straight. Keep the elbows at the sides, or even back a bit and the upper arm perpendicular to the floor. Pull the bar using just the biceps as far as possible without moving the elbows from the sides. Pause briefly at both ends of the movement. Make the initial pull very slow so you are not using momentum to move the weight. Do pure reps, smooth and slow.

2. Try to drag the bar along the front of the body, almost touching the body as it is pulled up. Do not bend the hand toward the body. Keep the wrist bent away from the body slightly.

OVERHEAD PRESS

1. Try to keep continuous tension on the shoulder muscles by stopping just short of a full extension of the arms, and then slowly lower the bar to the chest or the back of the neck. Pause for a second and press it overhead from a dead stop.

2. Keep the back straight.

3. Do the movement while seated to minimize the stress on the back.

CRUNCH SITUPS

1. Lie flat and bend the knees up toward the head. Curl your body like you are rolling up a carpet.

2. Hold each rep for a full second at the top of the movement. Do not lower your upper body all the way down. Stop just short of your upper body being fully extended, and curl yourself back up. Always try to keep the tension constant on the muscles by doing each rep slowly. It is important to start each rep slowly to better sense the action of the abdominal muscles.

3. Do not stabilize your feet by placing them under a pad or on a bar.

LEG EXTENSIONS

1. Place your hands on top of your thighs to feel the muscles contracting as you slowly straighten the leg. Hold the contraction at the top for a moment, and then lower the weight slowly. Pause briefly at the bottom of the rep but do not relax the muscle. As always, do smooth, slow reps.

2. Vary the position of the feet on the pad.

3. Point your toes away from your body.

POSITIVE AND NEGATIVE

A man who dares to waste one hour of time has not discovered the value of life.
~~~Charles Darwin

Each rep has a positive half and a negative half. The positive part is known as concentric and the negative is called the eccentric.

A muscle is working during both phases of the rep. When the muscle is working against gravity, it is the concentric part of the rep. When the muscle is resisting the pull of gravity, it is the eccentric part of the rep. Always control the rep through both parts of the movement to derive the maximum benefit from the rep. Don't do only the negative part of the rep. If you cannot do the positive part of the rep, stop your set.

SAFETY

It is health that is real wealth, and not pieces of gold and silver.

~~~Mahatma Gandhi

You will find that a major theme of this book is safety. Does it make sense that you should live a safe lifestyle? Does it make sense that living a risky and reckless life that has stupid behavior will only lead to problems?

When you get out of bed to start your day, do you tell yourself that you are going to drive to work recklessly in order to try to arrive in less time than yesterday? Of course you don't. You recognize such a behavior as unsafe, risky, and stupid. The goal is to arrive safely. The time to get there is irrelevant.

Do you get up in the morning and plan your meals to include unhealthy food? Do you eat and drink in a way that is not safe for your health, much the same as driving recklessly? Or do you create a diet plan that is safe for your health?

When you exercise, do you ignore the risk that is part of the process and use too much weight, in bad form, and with little control? Do you train in a way that is not safe for your body? Or do you acknowledge the risk, and exercise in a safe manner?

Be sensible. Live safely. Eat safely. Exercise safely. Preserve your body and your health.

FULL BODY OR SPLIT WORKOUT

Whether you think that you can, or that you can't, you are usually right.

~~~Henry Ford

Depending on the amount of time you have available to train, or the time you personally want to spend in the gym, you have several options regarding the structure of your workouts. A full body workout and a split routine are two options.

In a full body workout, you train the entire body at one session. A basic full body session may include one compound movement for each body part. Another might add an isolation movement before or after the compound movement, or use the isolation exercise alone. Whatever your decision is regarding the exercises you use, try to keep your rest time to a minimum. Train the larger muscle groups (legs, chest, and back) first in the workout. Work the adjoining muscle groups in sequence, i.e. chest and back, legs and calves, shoulders and arms. Keep the blood flow in the same area of the body.

The other option is a split routine. You divide the program into two- or three-day sections according to the body parts to be trained each day. The varieties are numerous. One option would be to do upper body one day, lower body another day. Another might be to do pushing movements one day and pulling movements another day.

Keep in mind that training the same joint area on consecutive days can lead to injury from overtraining. This is especially true of the shoulder and lower back. Experiment, but be sensible and in tune with your body.

Do not be rigid in your choice of exercises or programs. Train on a full body schedule for a while, and then try a split routine. Step outside the box, and enjoy your training by consistently giving your muscles and mind a variety of movements. Remember: keep your muscles confused. You will find it easier to create a congested feeling with a varied choice of exercises over time. Change the exercise to make unaccustomed work for your body to handle by adaptation, and therefore better progress in your training.

CIRCUIT TRAINING

The circuit training program along with a healthy clean diet is the way to excellent results.

~~~Lee Haney,

8x Mr. Olympia

Circuit training is a training technique that involves performing consecutive sets of exercises for different body parts without rest, then repeating the sequence. The method is also known as peripheral heart action, or PHA. Your use of the method may depend on the availability of equipment at the time you need it. The Universal gym machine, or any other multi-station exercise equipment, is ideal for a circuit training workout.

An example of a circuit or cycle of exercises would be squats, dips, chins, and dumbbell presses. Do a set of squats, followed immediately by a set of dips, followed immediately by a set of chins, and then a set of dumbbell presses for the entire cycle. Take only as much rest between the sets as is required to move to the equipment for the next exercise. After a brief rest, repeat the cycle a couple of times. Then do another cycle of different movements. This method of training provides an opportunity for creativity and variety, in addition to giving the total body a good cardiovascular workout.

COMPOUNDS SAVE TIME

It is far better to be alone, than to be in bad company.

~~~George Washington

Time is valuable, particularly when it is non-employment time. We all have our real world responsibilities outside of our employment, and often the time to do a training session is not easily available.

For time savings, do the compound movements available for each muscle group. A compound exercise will train several individual muscles simultaneously. Smaller muscles like the biceps and triceps benefit from the indirect effect of the compound movement. An example of a group of compound exercises that would comprise a quick session is:

Abdominal crunches

Leg press

Bench press

Lat machine pulldowns

Overhead dumbbell presses

This combination can be completed in a fairly short time, yet it has worked all the major muscle groups in your body.

CALVES

A man needs a purpose for real health.

~~~Sherwood Anderson

The calves can be difficult to improve because the muscles are subjected to the constant stress of walking. All day long, your calf muscles are extending your foot away from you or pointing your toes toward you against the resistance of your bodyweight. Further, genetically some people have inherited good calf muscles and some have not been so lucky.

The typical standing or seated calf raises are the basic exercises for this body part. Always do a full movement of the heel through the range of motion, up as high as possible, and down as low as possible. Stop and hold the contraction at the top, and do the movement slowly. Don't use too much weight.

FLEX BETWEEN SETS

Be happy for this moment. This moment is your life.

~~~Omar Khayyam

As inconspicuously as possible, flex the muscles you trained in the last set by tensing the muscle in its fully contracted position. This action will help to increase the sensory connection between your brain and the muscle tissue, thereby enhancing the ability to sense the congested feeling.

I recommend that you not imitate a peacock when flexing. Simply contract the muscle for a moment to get the sense of its presence in your body and the congestive effect of the exercise.

GRIP

The human body is the best picture of the human soul.

~~~Ludwig Wittgenstein

Most exercises for the upper body require you to grip a bar. Always grip as tightly as possible. A good grip gives your mind confidence and a sense of strength. When the grip is weak, your attention is diverted to losing your grasp.

Include some type of forearm exercise in your training. The grip is determined by the strength of the muscles in the forearm, so the results will enhance your ability to do other exercises effectively. Wrist curls with a barbell or dumbbells is the traditional exercise. Hold the bar with your hand bent back slightly and use the forearm muscles to bend the hand toward the forearm. Do the reps slowly and hold the bar in the fully contracted position. The forearms respond quickly to exercise, and the pump is easily sensed after a few sets of fairly high reps.

BACK EXERCISE

The discipline of desire is the background of character.
~~~John Locke

The function of the large back muscles called the latissimus dorsi (lats) is to pull the upper arm bone closer to the upper body. Most exercise movements for the lats also involve flexing the forearm toward the upper arm using the smaller biceps muscle to bend the arm against the resistance.

When doing chin ups or pulldowns on a pulley machine, vary your grip to change the effect of the exercise. Place your hands with palms facing away from you, toward you, or facing each other. You can also vary the spacing of the hands on the bar. You will change the effect the exercise has on the back and the indirect effect it has on the biceps.

Try to squeeze your shoulder blades together as the arms come closer to the body. Think about pulling your elbows down and back as opposed to pulling your arms. A word of caution: do not use an extremely wide grip, as it may damage your shoulders.

A good exercise to isolate the lats without using the biceps is straight arm pulldowns on the overhead pulley machine. Stand in front of the bar, grab it with your thumb on top of the bar and bend forward slightly at the waist. Keep your back straight and your head up. Without bending the arms, drag the bar to the thighs, hold it for a moment, and then slowly let it rise to the starting point. The movement is similar to a swimming stroke. Use a light weight for 12-20 reps.

I have found this exercise is good to isolate the lats in a pre-exhaustion routine. The "weak link" of the biceps is eliminated in pulling the bar by the lats. Do a set of straight-arm pulldowns followed by a set of regular pulldowns or chin ups for a good back pump.

POSTURE

Reputation is what men and women think of us; character is what God and angels know of us.

~~~Thomas Paine

Good posture is important in every exercise. When you keep the back straight (by flexing the big muscles in the back) and your shoulders up and back, you create a stronger foundation for doing the exercise and also decrease the chance of injury. Proper posture creates good body mechanics for the performance of an exercise.

Posture is also important outside the gym. Your appearance and the maintenance of your back depend on your choice of how you stand or sit, i.e. slouched or straight. It does not make sense to work hard to improve your health and appearance, but let your posture hide the results of your efforts or ruin your back.

ABDOMINAL MUSCLES AND LOWER BACK

A merry heart doeth good like a medicine, but a broken spirit dries the bones.

~~~Proverbs

Try to balance your development by working the antagonistic muscles that move bones in opposite directions. This is particularly true with the abdominal muscles and lower back. An imbalance in this area, particularly if due to less lower back strength relative to abdominal strength, can lead to problems.

Try doing an abdominal exercise followed by a lower back movement, alternating back and forth for 3-4 sets. For example, do a set of abdominal crunches followed by a set of hyperextensions. Keep the blood flowing to the area by taking little rest between the two sets.

Part Three

Diet

DON'T BE FOOLED

*The only way you get that fat off is to eat less and exercise
more.*
~~~Jack LaLanne

Do not let exercise fool you into thinking that training
alone is the most important factor in improving your health,
appearance, and fitness. You must have a balance of
exercise and good dietary habits, but ultimately your choice
of food and drink will be a bigger factor than your choice
of exercises. Training hard followed by overindulging in
food and drink does you no good. You are engaging in a
self-defeating and unsafe cycle of compensatory exercise
and dereliction. You can't run faster than your fork.

Training regularly is certainly a good habit to acquire,
but your decisions regarding food and drink will have a
greater effect on your appearance and health. Frankly, the
best exercise for losing weight is the push away. Just push
yourself away from the table when you are no longer
hungry.

KEEP IT SMALL

We never repent of having eaten too little.

~~~Thomas Jefferson

An old maxim in bodybuilding is that if you want something to be small, don't put much into it. This philosophy is especially true in the old adage that the eyes are sometimes bigger than the stomach.

Physiologically and anatomically the concept is very simple. The abdominal area has the ability to expand in order to accommodate the quantity of food and drink that is stored in the stomach after a meal. Given the fact that the stomach area normally is the size of your fist, you can see that it does not take much food or liquid to fill a cavity that size. Simple equation: more = big, and less = small.

Eat several small meals daily to avoid bloating the stomach. If your training time is after work, eat something prior to your workout so that your blood sugar level and energy are high enough to support the exercise.

The less you put into your body at one time, the more efficiently your body uses it. Don't keep eating until you are full; instead, eat until you do not feel hungry. If you are in tune with your body, you will lose your feeling of hunger long before you feel full of food and drink. Nibble food and sip drinks over the course of the day.

BOX IT UP

He who has a why to live for can bear almost any how.

~~~Nietzsche

When dining out, a restaurant is likely to serve more than you can comfortably consume at one time. Anticipate when you sit at the table that you are going to purchase two meals. Slowly eat a portion of the meal (until you sense you are no longer hungry) and take the rest home in a box. You get two meals for the price of one, and you avoid overloading the digestive system.

Ask for a box when you order your food. Let the box sitting on the table serve as your reminder to stop eating while there is still food on your plate. Don't let the menu or the portion sizes dictate your eating pattern. Common sense goes a long way toward healthy living.

EAT UNTIL YOU ARE NOT HUNGRY

In general, mankind, since the improvement of cookery,
eats twice as much as nature requires.

~~~Benjamin Franklin

Once food is in the stomach, there is little sensory input to the brain regarding its presence. The smooth muscle tissue in the digestive tract does not have the sensory system to tell you what is happening as food moves through it. There is no good reason to have that sense. The only sense that exists is when the stomach is storing excess food and liquid, causing the abdominal area to expand. This creates a bloated and uncomfortable feeling.

Learn to sense this feeling when it happens. Think of it as being uncomfortable, and avoid it by slowly consuming smaller amounts of food and liquid at one time. Stop eating when you begin to feel that you are no longer hungry, which should be well before your stomach is filled to capacity. It is better to feel no hunger than to be stuffed full of excess food and liquid. Instead of saying, "I'm full" as the reason to stop eating, get into the habit of saying, "I'm no longer hungry."

There are some stimuli to our sensory system that are easy to feel and some that are more difficult to feel. For example, it is not difficult to sense that you are cold and need to put on a coat for warmth. In the same way, you should be able to sense that you are no longer hungry and need to stop eating.

BE A NIBBLER

Our bodies are our gardens—our wills are our gardeners.
~~~William Shakespeare

Acquire the habit of eating several small meals throughout the day. You will not overload the digestive system, thereby creating more efficient breakdown, absorption, and assimilation of food. The body cannot properly digest food if you put too much into it. Equally important, you will avoid expansion of the abdomen. The less you eat at one time, the more efficiently your body is able to use what you put into it. Nibble periodically throughout the day as your eating habit. Be a grazer.

Think of it as if you are working on an assembly line. If your foreman did not give you much work until the end of the day, and then gave you an entire day's worth to do in a short time, you would not be able to do the work as efficiently as if the work was parceled out in smaller amounts throughout the day.

When you eat too much at one time, you simply feel lousy. You become lethargic and bloated, feeling like the only thing you want to do is lay down and rest. Overeating saps your vitality and energy. The same feeling would overcome you on the assembly line. Too much work at one time would leave you depressed and uncomfortable with your ability to handle it.

Some people have the habit of filling a glass completely, or filling a plate with food. Does it make sense to let the size of the glass or the size of the plate determine the quantity you consume? Try using a smaller glass and plate to decrease the amount you are consuming.

A study was done on rats in which one group was given three meals a day and the second group was allowed to nibble all day. At the end of the experiment, the rats in both groups weighed about the same. However, the rats in the first group had more body fat than the rats that nibbled at their food. The better strategy is to be a nibbler and not a meal eater. You will never be hungry and you will never be full.

EAT AND DRINK SLOWLY

Health is the greatest gift, contentment the greatest wealth, faithfulness the best relationship.

~~~Buddha

You should develop the habit of eating slowly and chewing food to the point where you almost do not have to swallow it. This habit serves three purposes:

1. You sense the taste of the food more.
2. The process makes it easier for the rest of the digestive system to finish breaking the food down for absorption.
3. You will eat less at one sitting because the time spent will give you the opportunity to sense that you are no longer hungry.

My great-grandfather would take an hour to eat dinner. I do not think his dining habit was unique to his era. Most of the time was spent chatting among the family, and not eating. Dinner was the only time of the day when the family was together. The benefit of this habit has long been recognized as beneficial to health.

Put your fork down between bites. Eat slowly. Stop eating before the food is gone and ask yourself if you are still hungry. No one is going to take the food away from you.

Sip your drinks instead of gulping down a large quantity. You overload your stomach and create a bloated feeling. Drinking slowly permits your body to deal with the liquid gradually and more effectively. Minimize the quantity of liquid you consume with a meal so you do not bloat your stomach.

ROCKS

When men speak ill of thee, live so as nobody may believe them.

~~~Plato

When I was growing up in Ohio, our family business was asphalt blacktop paving of driveways and parking lots. An important part of the job was working with gravel to create a solid base to spread the asphalt.

I recall there were two types of gravel that we used. One was called "3D" and was basically large rocks the size of tennis balls. The other was "46D" and was a mix of much smaller rocks and a sandy mixture made from grinding up the rocks.

The gravel was dumped into piles and our job was to use shovels to spread the piles out as evenly as possible so it could be raked and rolled as a level surface for paving. We used long-handled shovels with spade shaped blades.

Shoveling the 46D was not that difficult. The gravel was ground into a fine, loose mixture and the shovel lifted it easily.

The 3D gravel was a different story. The larger rocks were incredibly difficult to separate and lift with the shovel. The job took much more effort than dealing with the smaller gravel. We did not enjoy working with the 3D gravel.

Think of chewing your food in the same way that I described my experience on the blacktop crew. Shoveling the smaller gravel was easier than the larger rocks. Your body finds it much easier to break down, digest and assimilate food that has been thoroughly chewed into an almost liquid consistency. If you don't chew food and instead swallow it in large pieces, your digestive system gets stressed trying to break it down and digest it. Even though you cannot feel it, your body is working hard to deal with the unchewed food.

Think of my blacktop job when you are eating. Give your body some easy 46D food to deal with instead of difficult 3D food chunks.

SENSE YOUR GUT

A sound mind in a sound body is a short but full description of a happy state in this world.

~~~John Locke

There are two points in the digestive process that involve a sense or feeling of what is happening with the food and drink you ingest. The first is in the mouth, and the second is in the abdomen. Most people focus on the stimulating sensory feeling that the taste of food gives them and ignore the feeling created in the abdomen by the process of filling the stomach area of the system.

The stomach portion of the digestive tract normally is the size of your fist when empty. It narrows into a small valve-like opening which controls the flow of food out of the stomach area, thereby permitting it to remain in the stomach for better breakdown. This small space is not much room for food and liquid.

Do not consume an amount of food or drink that exceeds the storage capacity of the stomach. Do not ignore the sense of fullness in the abdomen caused by the normal expansion of the stomach as it fills with food and liquid. You should not eat so much that it forces the abdominal area to expand to accommodate the volume.

Pay the most attention to the sense created in the abdominal area when you eat, and stop when you are no longer hungry. Enjoy the taste of food by chewing thoroughly, but do not continue to eat more than you need just to prolong the sensory stimulation in the mouth. Satisfy your body's needs and not your artificial cravings. Your priority should be to sense your stomach, not your taste buds. The taste sensation is a short term effect. Flavor selection is a poor method of safe eating.

Your body's health should be your long term goal. If you wait until you feel that your stomach is full, you have waited too long to stop eating. Know when to stop. As the book of Proverbs says, "A wise man eats to live; a fool lives to eat."

POOR EATING PATTERN

He who drinks and has no thirst,
Like he who eats and has no hunger,
Unlike he whose health is first,
Suffers illness and dies younger.

~~~Swami Sivananda

When it comes to a choice of food and the quantity eaten, many people exhibit poor discipline in the morning and in the evening. For some reason, breakfast is the meal where it is easier to eat less or nothing at all. Many of us feel we have insufficient time to prepare for work and also have a good breakfast. Then at night, the feeling that we have earned the right to overeat or eat the wrong foods takes over, and a regrettable overindulgence occurs.

I think that people avoid eating a decent breakfast because they are afraid of having to consciously sense the feeling of fullness in the stomach throughout the day. If an excess has been consumed, the feeling is an uncomfortable distraction and negatively impacts the ability to focus on a daily activity. Just think how difficult it is to work after eating a large lunch.

Dinner is a different situation. Food becomes a comfort and a sensual part of the end of the day, indeed a reward of sorts, instead of simply serving the function of providing nutrition and energy. You can overindulge, then sit and do a whole lot of nothing for the rest of the evening, without having to truly function in a productive manner with a bloated stomach. When you do not have to deal with it, it is not noticeable.

191

Another reason for this eating pattern is the false sense people have that they are actually dieting for weight loss by following poor nutritional support during the day. They are foolishly thinking that they are consuming fewer calories, notwithstanding the fact that they eat a heavy meal at night. Further, by eating too much at night, they will not feel truly hungry in the morning, thus perpetuating the cycle.

Rather than consuming the bulk of your calories at dinner, try to "graze" throughout the day, mixing lighter meals with healthy snacks in between. Then, after a light dinner, avoid further eating. If you find it difficult to stop snacking in the evening, try brushing your teeth immediately after dinner.

If you are limited to three meals a day, eat like a king at breakfast, a prince at lunch, and a pauper at dinner. This pattern is consistent with the decreasing need for energy throughout the day. You may also find that eating less at night just makes you feel better. Do not be afraid of waking up feeling hungry. Why do you think it is called break-fast?

REAL FOOD

Man seeks to change the foods available in nature to suit his tastes, thereby putting an end to the very essence of life contained in them.

~~~Sai Baba

There are an infinite number of food choices. Mankind has been making decisions about food and drink for thousands of years. Our bodies have adapted to assimilate, absorb, and survive on the food that has been available during that time period.

Consider the fact that many of the food choices available today are essentially man-made virtual food, as opposed to the foods made by nature over thousands of years. Virtual food is artificial and foreign to our body chemistry, and is "processed" to make it more commercially profitable.

Our bodies are accustomed to using living, natural food for growth and energy. This concept is not rocket science. You learned the basics in health class. Eat some food from the basic groups (dairy, meat, fruit, vegetables, and grains) in its natural form.

Read the ingredients on a box of food. Note the names of chemicals compared with food. My guess is that the ingredients are not familiar to you, yet you are choosing to add those chemicals to your body. Calcium carbonate, tripotassium phosphate, maltodextrin, yellow 5 lake, yellow 6 lake, and sodium bisulfite are not exactly as well-known as an apple or an orange, but whatever those chemicals are and whatever effect they may have on your body should be taken into consideration when you choose to eat processed food. Would you go to a chemical supply store and purchase these ingredients to eat individually?

In a nutshell, if nature did not make it, do not eat it. Eat safely.

THE JAW

Believe nothing, no matter where you read it or who said it—even if I said it—unless it agrees with your own reason and your own common sense.

~~~Buddha

When was the last time you saw a person with his or her mandible (jawbone) visible? To put it another way, observe the people around you who have excess tissue extending from the chin to the throat like a goiter, or a wattle on a turkey. No jaw line is visible, and the entire face is distorted from the front and the side. Do you think that a double or triple chin, as such a condition is called, has become the norm today? How would such a person's facial features appear with a visible jawbone?

One of the first things you notice if you compare a photo from the teenage years with a photo many years later is the change in facial appearance caused by fat accumulation. If you lose weight throughout the entire body, you lose weight in the face as well. When was the last time you saw your jaw? Are your facial features defined by fat tissue? Do you like it?

SPONGE THEORY

He who takes medicine and neglects to his diet wastes the skill of his doctors.

~~~Chinese Proverb

Think of your body as a large sponge. Like a sponge, your body absorbs what you choose to put into it. Put water into a sponge and it expands with the absorption and gets heavy. Squeeze the sponge so as to remove the water and it gets smaller and lighter.

If you put too much food and drink into the body, it will expand like the sponge. By reducing your intake, your "sponge" will decrease in size. Also, like a sponge, your body will not discriminate between good things to absorb and bad things to absorb. The decision on what will be absorbed is yours. Practice wise selective absorption of healthy food and drink.

CALORIES

Worthless people live only to eat and drink; people of
worth eat and drink only to live.

~~~Socrates

The energy content of all food is measured in terms of calories. Some foods have more calories than others, and are thus capable of providing more energy. Calories which are not used are stored as fat. The equation is simple. If calories consumed exceed calories expended, over time you will gain weight. If calories consumed are less than calories expended, over time you will lose weight.

Study the calorie content of the foods and drinks you consume. Read the labels and compare calories. You may find that, generally, natural foods like fruits and vegetables contain fewer calories than man-made or processed foods. A diet that is made up of natural foods will be low in calories but high in nutritional value.

Avoid foods that have concentrated calories. By this I mean food that has a high calorie density, i.e. a large number of calories in a small portion, like candy and other foods with sugar.

Think of calories in the opposite manner that you think of money management. You cannot spend more money than you earn. You cannot consume more calories than you use for energy without gaining fat body weight. Eat a maintenance diet if you are satisfied with your appearance.

NO SALT

Walking is the best possible exercise. Habituate yourself to walk very far.

~~~Thomas Jefferson

Do not add salt to your food and avoid foods with sodium. Salt will bloat your body with excess water. Sodium intake may also increase your blood pressure.

Check the labels on cans and packages of food to determine their sodium level. Notice that often the salt content will be given for only a small portion of the contents of the package. You may have to do some math to determine the entire sodium content for the package. Try to avoid those foods that are high in their sodium content.

FOOD IS COMFORT

Natural forces within us are the true healers of disease.
~~~Hippocrates

Food is a comfort to some people. There are many emotional aspects of our lives that are attached to our eating. Mealtime is often associated with fond memories of Mom, love, family, and a familiar pattern of behavior. So many memories include food: holiday dinners, birthday cakes, feeding our children. Food is associated with many emotions and habits that signify a common bond among those who have gathered to eat together.

Perhaps your mother or grandmother prepared your meals, particularly the evening meal. Was she, in her own loving way, somewhat pushy when it came to "encouraging" you to eat the food she prepared? Did you feel a bit pressured to eat past the point of your hunger disappearing by cleaning your plate? Did you learn to ignore the feeling of fullness in your stomach, and instead become more concerned with pleasing your mother by over eating? Did this emotional attitude develop and become a habit that has lasted throughout your life? Are you reluctant to change from this old habit? Why? Is your mother still being a bit pushy, if only in your mind?

You have to define your own individual nutritional needs, and satisfy those needs. Do not force feed yourself or eat because of stress. You should not cook more food than you need for a healthy meal. Avoid making gluttony a psychological distraction in your life. Eat only what you need and define your consumption by answering the question, "What do I need to eat?"

If you still find yourself looking for ways to get pleasure from your food, focus on planning healthy, varied meals, rather than on the act of eating itself. Enjoy the knowledge that, by changing your eating habits, you are doing something good for your body.

LOOK AROUND YOU

Strength of mind rests in sobriety; for this keeps your reason unclouded by passion.

~~~Pythagoras

In addition to taking a good look at yourself, check out the people around you and describe what you see. Objectively examine and evaluate the variety of physical appearances on display in your world. Note the number of people you see who are too heavy in proportion to their height and body frame. Also, note the people suffering from "done lap disease," i.e. their belly done lapped over their belt.

How many people do you observe with large abdomens, bloated faces, and excess weight? Note the number of people you see who are too thin for their height or body frame. What is the ratio of too-thin people to too-large people? Finally, how many people do you see who you would describe as lean or fit? What is the ratio of fit physiques to overweight physiques? Would you conclude that lean and fit people are the exception rather than the rule? No doubt the number of people you see on a daily basis who are too heavy in proportion to their height or body frame greatly exceeds the number of thin or fit persons.

Imagine that another person is doing the same evaluation of your body. Would you be considered too heavy? Too thin? Lean and fit? Are you proud of the category you think you would be placed in by another person? Which do you want to be?

In doing your evaluation of other people, ask yourself, "How did that person live his/her life in order to acquire the physical appearance I see?" Remember, it is no accident. If overweight, he or she was not born that way. An unsafe life of gluttony and overindulgence is readily apparent.

When I was 11 years old, I was an overweight fellow. Our family had a habit of overeating, particularly at dinner, and this was compounded by a nightly bowl of ice cream while watching television. The idea of healthy eating was not a concern with many people during that time period.

One evening I was at the bowling alley watching my father and grandfather bowl in a league. A good friend of my grandfather's, Cliff Robling, asked me to take a look at a fellow who was grossly obese. He must have weighed 350 pounds. Cliff told me "If you keep eating like you do now, that is how you will look in a few years." His frankness did not affect me to make a change at that time but the example he pointed out has remained with me since then.

What will you choose to imitate? Will it be a lifestyle of excess food and drink, and therefore excess weight and poor health? Or will you choose a safe lifestyle of sensible choices of quantity and quality of food and drink, exercise, and therefore better health and appearance? The people you see made decisions to follow a path of behavior to get where they are in terms of their appearance and health. What is your decision about yourself?

DIET

Everything in excess is opposed to nature.

~~~Hippocrates

The word "diet" is misleading, because it is generally used in the context of denial of something that is desirable. "On a diet" implies that someone is restricting themselves from eating particular foods that otherwise would be consumed. But your "diet" is really the choice of food and drink you make on a daily basis.

Focus on your diet as a positive, not a negative. Acquire the habit of selective food choice, both quality and quantity. The question should not be "What do I want to eat?" The question should be "What do I need to eat?" Eat foods that are beneficial to you and avoid those that are not. Stress natural, unprocessed food and avoid unnatural, changed food. Know the value of what you are eating.

Don't have the habit of indiscriminate eating, paying no real attention to what and how much you are putting into your body. Focus on the eating decisions you are making, and tell yourself you are making good decisions in your diet. Do not do something wrong for yourself. Do something right for yourself.

We are born with faculties and powers capable of almost anything, such as at least would carry us further than can be easily imagined: but it is only the exercise of those powers which gives us the ability and skill in anything, and leads us towards perfection.

~~~John Locke

To enjoy good health, to bring true happiness to one's family, to bring peace to all, one must first discipline and control one's mind.
If a man can control his mind he can find the way to enlightenment, and all wisdom and virtue will naturally come to him.

~~~Buddha

Regularity in the hours of rising and retiring, perseverance in exercise, adaptation of dress to the variations of climate, simple and nutritious aliment, and temperance in all things are necessary branches in the regime of health

~~~Lord Chesterfield

ABOUT THE AUTHOR

Bob Hoyle began weight training in 1966. He graduated from Harvard College in Cambridge, Massachusetts in 1975 with a degree in Biology. While at Harvard he wrestled and worked as a weight training instructor for the Harvard Department of Athletics.

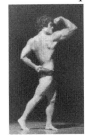 After graduating Bob decided to use his knowledge of weight training to benefit high school athletes. He taught high school biology and coached weightlifting, football and wrestling.

In his last year of coaching, his weightlifting team placed 4th in the Florida State High School Championships, and he also had one state champion lifter.

Bob competed in bodybuilding and powerlifting contests from 1971-1978. A shoulder injury forced him to give up those sports.

He graduated from Capital University Law School in Columbus, Ohio in 1986, and practices law in Bradenton, Florida. Bob published three articles in Iron Man Magazine: "How Much Can You Control," "A Basic Building Exercise," and "Try Parallel Bar Dips for Upper Body Development."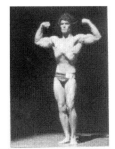

Bob lives in Bradenton, Florida, where he enjoys the relaxed Florida lifestyle.

Made in the USA
Charleston, SC
27 October 2015